The Complete Easy Metabolism Diet Meal Prep:

2024 Edition

"Boost Your Metabolism: The Complete Guide with Delicious Recipes and a 7-Day Customizable Meal Plan for Weight Loss"

Liam Bryce

1

TABLE OF CONTENTS:

INTRODUCTION

There was a vivacious woman named Eva who lived in the busy metropolis of New Hope. A devoted nurse, Eva had prioritized the needs of others before her health and well-being. Her weight increased, her energy levels decreased, and her once-sparkling eyes became duller with time. The world of nutrition and diets felt like a never-ending maze, even though she knew something had to change.

One day, as Eva sipped her cold coffee in the hospital break room, she heard her coworkers gushing about "The Complete Easy Metabolism Diet Meal Prep: 2024 Edition," a book that had completely changed their lives. She picked up the book out of curiosity and opened it, not thinking that this would be the first step toward becoming a happier, healthier version of herself.

Eva had never read a book quite like this one. It was more than simply a cookbook; it opened her eyes to the right nourishment of her body and its demands. The basic but effective idea behind the metabolism diet was to increase the body's innate capacity to burn fat by consuming the correct foods at the proper times. Without the limitations of rigid diets, it promised energy, weight loss, and a revitalized sense of vigor.

Equipped with her recently acquired information, Eva set out on her meal prep quest. She was astounded by the book's ability to simplify intricate dietary facts into simple-to-follow advice. In addition to being delicious, the meals were made to speed up her metabolism. Every meal was a step toward a healthier Emily, from the flavorful lemon-garlic salmon to the filling quinoa and black bean salad.

The changes in Eva were evident as the weeks stretched into months. She experienced a surge of energy, glowing skin, and a renewed sense of delight in taking care of herself. After noticing, friends and coworkers inquired about her secret. Eva would answer simply and with a smile, "It's all about the power of the right foods and a little bit of meal prep magic."

The Complete Easy Diet for Metabolism Meal Prep: 2024 Edition was as more than just a book for Eva; it was a traveling companion that helped her restore her vigor and health. It showed her that looking after oneself was necessary rather than selfish. As Eva began a new chapter in her life, she realized that she could create a narrative that was full of vitality, happiness, and well-being.

"The Complete Easy Metabolism Diet Meal Prep: 2024 Edition," your go-to resource for easily and deliciously improving your health, speeding up your metabolism, and reaching your weight loss objectives. This book is meant to make the process of becoming a more vibrant, energetic, and leaner version of yourself easier in a world when time is valuable and health is crucial.

Explore a variety of painstakingly created dishes that are not only delicious but also designed to increase metabolism and encourage fat-burning. Every meal is a step closer to your wellness goals than the last since every dish is the ideal combination of nutrients that work together to ignite your body's inherent fat-burning powers.

In addition to recipes, this edition is full of useful advice on meal planning that will help you make healthy eating not just a possibility but a fun and sustainable part of your everyday routine. This book is your road map to a more active and satisfying life, regardless of whether you're a working professional, a devoted parent, or just someone trying to take charge of your health.

With the help of "The Complete Easy Metabolism Diet Meal Prep: 2024 Edition," embrace the path to a more vibrant you. Bid farewell to conjecture and welcome to a future full of energy, self-assurance, and a metabolism that functions in your favor rather than against you. Together, let's go on this delightful trip.

Understanding Metabolism and Its Impact on Weight Loss

Understanding metabolism and its impact on weight loss is crucial for anyone looking to manage their weight effectively. The intricate metabolic reactions that take place inside our bodies to transform food and liquids into energy are referred to as metabolism. This energy is used for various bodily functions, such as breathing, circulating blood, and cell repair.

Basal Metabolic Rate (BMR)

A significant component of metabolism is the basal metabolic rate (BMR), which accounts for the number of calories your body needs to perform basic life-sustaining functions. Factors that influence BMR include age, sex, body composition, and genetics. Generally, a higher muscle mass leads to a higher BMR, as muscles are more metabolically active than fat.

Metabolism and Weight Loss

When it comes to weight loss, metabolism plays a pivotal role. If your body burns more calories than it consumes, you will lose weight. You will, on the other hand, acquire weight if you eat more calories than your body expels. This is where the concept of "energy balance" comes into play.

Boosting Metabolism for Weight Loss

Increase Muscle Mass: Engaging in strength training exercises can help build muscle, which in turn can increase your BMR and enhance calorie burning.

Eat Protein-Rich Foods: Protein has a higher thermic effect than carbohydrates or fats, meaning your body burns more calories digesting protein. Incorporating protein into your meals can boost metabolism and reduce appetite.

Stay Hydrated: Drinking water can temporarily speed up metabolism. Cold water is even more effective, as your body uses energy to heat it to body temperature.

Eat Small, Frequent Meals: Eating small, frequent meals throughout the day can keep your metabolism active, preventing it from slowing down between meals.

Get Enough Sleep: Get Enough Sleep: Sleep deprivation can accelerate weight gain by impairing metabolism. Ensuring adequate sleep is essential for maintaining a healthy metabolic rate.

Manage Stress: Chronic stress can lead to hormonal imbalances that may slow down metabolism. Engaging in stress-reducing activities like meditation or yoga can help keep your metabolism in check.

Understanding metabolism and its impact on weight loss is essential for anyone looking to manage their weight effectively. By making lifestyle changes that boost metabolism, such as increasing muscle mass, eating protein-rich foods, staying hydrated, eating small frequent meals, getting enough sleep, and managing stress, you can enhance your body's ability to burn calories and achieve your weight loss goals.

The Principles of the Metabolism Diet

The Metabolism Diet is based on the principle of optimizing your body's natural metabolic processes to achieve weight loss and improve overall health. Here are some key principles that underpin this diet:

Eat the Right Foods at the Right Times: The Metabolism Diet emphasizes the importance of not only what you eat but also when you eat. It encourages consuming meals that kick-start your metabolism at specific times of the day to keep it running efficiently.

Balance Macronutrients: This diet focuses on balancing carbohydrates, proteins, and fats in each meal to provide steady energy and prevent spikes in blood sugar levels. This balance helps in maintaining a healthy metabolic rate.

Frequent, Small Meals: Instead of three large meals, the Metabolism Diet recommends eating five to six smaller meals throughout the day. This approach is believed to keep the metabolism active and prevent it from slowing down.

Hydration: Staying well-hydrated is crucial in the Metabolism Diet, as water is essential for various metabolic processes. Drinking adequate water can also help in suppressing appetite and preventing overeating.

Limit Processed Foods and Sugars: The diet advises limiting the intake of processed foods, refined sugars, and unhealthy fats, which can negatively impact metabolism and lead to weight gain.

Incorporate Metabolism-Boosting Foods: Certain foods are known to boost metabolism, such as lean proteins, spicy foods, green tea, and foods rich in omega-3 fatty acids. The Metabolism Diet includes these foods to enhance metabolic rate.

Regular Exercise: Physical activity is an integral part of the Metabolism Diet. Regular exercise, especially strength training and high-intensity interval training (HIIT), can increase muscle mass and boost metabolism.

Adequate Sleep: Getting enough quality sleep is essential for a healthy metabolism. The diet emphasizes the importance of sleep in regulating hormones that control hunger and metabolism.

Stress Management: Chronic stress can negatively affect metabolism. The Metabolism Diet encourages practices like meditation, yoga, or deep breathing exercises to manage stress levels.

Personalization: The diet recognizes that each individual's metabolic rate and nutritional needs are different. It encourages personalization of the diet plan based on one's unique body composition, lifestyle, and health goals.

By following these principles, the Metabolism Diet aims to optimize metabolic function, promote fat burning, and support sustainable weight loss and overall well-being.

The Benefits of Meal Prepping for Metabolic Health

Meal prepping, the practice of planning and preparing meals in advance, offers numerous benefits for metabolic health, making it a valuable habit for anyone looking to optimize their metabolism and maintain a healthy weight. Here are some key benefits of meal prepping for metabolic health:

Consistent Nutrient Intake: Meal prepping ensures that you have balanced meals with the right mix of macronutrients (carbohydrates, proteins, and fats) and micronutrients (vitamins and minerals) readily available. Consistent intake of these nutrients is crucial for maintaining a healthy metabolism.

Portion Control: Preparing meals in advance allows you to control portion sizes, which can help prevent overeating and promote weight management. Portion control is essential for regulating calorie intake, a key factor in metabolic health.

Reduced Reliance on Processed Foods: Meal prepping encourages the use of whole, unprocessed foods, which are generally lower in added sugars, unhealthy fats, and artificial additives that can negatively impact metabolism.

Better Blood Sugar Management: By having balanced meals prepared ahead of time, you can prevent large fluctuations in blood sugar levels, which is important for metabolic health and reducing the higher likelihood of developing insulin resistance and type 2 diabetes.

Time Efficiency: Meal prepping saves time in the long run, reducing the likelihood of resorting to fast food or convenience meals that are often high in calories and low in nutrients. This can contribute to a healthier diet overall.

Stress Reduction: Knowing that your meals are planned and prepared in advance can reduce stress and decision fatigue related to meal choices. Lower stress levels are beneficial for metabolic health, as chronic stress can disrupt metabolic processes.

Improved Digestive Health: Regular consumption of home-cooked, nutrient-dense meals can support gut health, which is closely linked to metabolic health. A healthy gut microbiome can aid in digestion, nutrient absorption, and regulation of metabolism.

Enhanced Hydration: Meal prepping often involves planning for beverages as well, encouraging the inclusion of hydrating drinks like water, herbal teas, or infused water. Proper hydration is essential for various metabolic processes in the body.

Customization for Specific Needs: Meal prepping allows for customization of meals to cater to individual dietary needs, preferences, and metabolic goals, whether it's low-carb, high-protein, or plant-based.

Increased Accountability: Having meals prepared in advance increases accountability and commitment to a healthy eating plan, which can lead to more consistent dietary habits and improved metabolic health over time.

Incorporating meal prepping into your routine can be a powerful tool for enhancing metabolic health, supporting weight management, and promoting overall well-being.

GETTING STARTED WITH METABOLISM DIET MEAL PREP

Essential Kitchen Tools and Equipment

When following a metabolic diet, having the right kitchen tools and equipment can make meal preparation easier and more efficient. Some essential items to consider:

Food Scale: A food scale is crucial for portion control and ensuring accurate measurements of ingredients, which is important for maintaining the balance of macronutrients in your meals.

Measuring Cups and Spoons: These are essential for measuring ingredients, especially when following specific recipes that require precise quantities to maintain the nutritional balance of your meals.

Blender or Food Processor: A high-quality blender or food processor is useful for making smoothies, soups, sauces, and purees that are common in metabolic diets.

Non-Stick Cookware: Non-stick pots and pans allow for cooking with less oil, which is beneficial for preparing low-fat meals that are often recommended in a metabolic diet.

Steamer Basket or Steamer Pot: Steaming is a healthy cooking method that preserves nutrients in vegetables and proteins, making a steamer an important tool for preparing metabolic-friendly meals.

Slow Cooker or Pressure Cooker: These appliances are great for preparing lean proteins and legumes, which are staples in a metabolic diet. They allow for convenient, hands-off cooking, making it easier to prepare healthy meals.

Glass Storage Containers: Having a set of glass storage containers is essential for meal prepping and storing leftovers. They are durable, microwave-safe, and don't retain odors or stains.

Sharp Knives: A set of sharp knives is necessary for efficient food preparation, whether you're chopping vegetables, slicing meat, or mincing herbs.

Cutting Boards: Invest in a few good-quality cutting boards to protect your countertops and ensure a safe and hygienic surface for food preparation.

Mixing Bowls: A variety of mixing bowls in different sizes is useful for mixing ingredients, marinating proteins, and assembling salads.

Salad Spinner: A salad spinner is helpful for washing and drying leafy greens, which are often a significant part of a metabolic diet.

Citrus Juicer or Zester: These tools are useful for adding flavor to dishes without extra calories, which is important for metabolic diet recipes.

Spice Grinder: A spice grinder allows you to grind fresh spices, which can enhance the flavor of your meals without adding sodium or sugar.

Digital Thermometer: A digital thermometer is essential for ensuring that meats are cooked to the proper temperature, which is important for both food safety and quality.

Baking Sheets and Parchment Paper: These are useful for roasting vegetables and proteins, a common cooking method in metabolic diet recipes.

Having these essential kitchen tools and equipment can help you efficiently prepare meals that align with the principles of a metabolic diet, making it easier to stick to your health and wellness goals.

Pantry Staples for Metabolic Cooking

Stocking your pantry with the right staples is key to successful metabolic cooking. These ingredients support a diet focused on boosting metabolism and promoting overall health. Here are some essential pantry staples for metabolic cooking:

- Whole Grains: Quinoa, brown rice, oats, and barley provide complex carbohydrates and fiber, which are important for sustained energy and digestive health.

- Legumes: Lentils, chickpeas, black beans, and kidney beans are excellent sources of plant-based protein and fiber, supporting metabolism and satiety.

- Nuts and Seeds: Almonds, walnuts, chia seeds, flaxseeds, and pumpkin seeds offer healthy fats, protein, and fiber, all of which are beneficial for metabolic health.

- Spices and Herbs: Cinnamon, turmeric, ginger, cayenne pepper, and fresh herbs like basil and parsley can boost flavor and metabolism without adding calories.

- Healthy Oils: Extra virgin olive oil, avocado oil, and coconut oil provide healthy fats that are essential for hormone production and nutrient absorption.

- Vinegars and Citrus: Apple cider vinegar, balsamic vinegar, lemons, and limes add flavor to dishes and can aid in digestion and blood sugar regulation.

- Low-Sodium Broths: Vegetable, chicken, or bone broths are great for soups and stews, providing hydration and nutrients while keeping sodium intake in check.

- Natural Sweeteners: Raw honey, maple syrup, and stevia are better alternatives to refined sugars for adding sweetness to recipes.

- Canned Goods: Canned tomatoes, pumpkin puree, and coconut milk are convenient for making sauces, soups, and curries.

- Whole Grain or Gluten-Free Pasta: Options like whole wheat, brown rice, or chickpea pasta offer a healthier alternative to traditional white pasta.

- Protein Powders: Whey, pea, or hemp protein powders can be added to smoothies or baked goods for an extra protein boost.

- Tea and Coffee: Green tea and black coffee are rich in antioxidants and can help boost metabolism when consumed in moderation.

- Dried Fruits: Unsweetened dried fruits like apricots, dates, and raisins can be used as natural sweeteners or snacks.

- Dark Chocolate: High-quality dark chocolate with a high cocoa content is a delicious treat that offers antioxidants and can support heart health.

- Nut Butters: Almond butter, peanut butter, and other nut butters are great for adding healthy fats and protein to snacks and meals.

Having these pantry staples on hand makes it easier to prepare meals that align with the principles of metabolic cooking, supporting your health and wellness goals.

Tips for Efficient and Effective Meal Prepping

Meal prepping can be a game-changer for maintaining a metabolic diet, ensuring that you have healthy, metabolism-boosting meals ready when you need them. Here are some tips for efficient and effective meal prepping:

- Organize Your Meals: To begin, you should organize your meals for the upcoming week. Consider your schedule and choose recipes that fit your metabolic diet goals. In order to guarantee that you have all of the required components, you should create a shopping list based on your meal plan.

- Batch Cook: Cook large batches of staple ingredients like grains, legumes, and proteins at the beginning of the week. Store them in the fridge or freezer, so you can easily assemble meals throughout the week.

- Prep Ingredients: Wash, chop, and portion out vegetables and fruits. Store them in airtight containers in the fridge for easy access when cooking or assembling meals.

- Use Versatile Ingredients: Choose ingredients that can be used in multiple recipes throughout the week. For example, cooked chicken can be used in salads, wraps, and stir-fries.

- Invest in Quality Containers: Use microwave-safe, freezer-safe, and leak-proof containers to store your prepped meals and ingredients. Glass containers are a great option as they are durable and don't retain odors.

- Label Your Containers: Label your containers with the contents and the date you prepared them. This will help you keep track of what's in your fridge and ensure you use ingredients while they're fresh.

- Schedule a Prep Day: Set aside a few hours on a designated day each week to do your meal prep. This will save you time and effort during the busy weekdays.

- Keep It Simple: Don't overcomplicate your meal prep. Stick to simple recipes and ingredients that you enjoy and that fit your metabolic diet plan.

- Include Snacks: Prep healthy snacks like cut-up vegetables, nuts, and yogurt to have on hand for when you need a quick energy boost.

- Stay Hydrated: Don't forget to include beverages in your meal prep. Prepare infused waters or herbal teas to ensure you stay hydrated throughout the week.

By following these tips, you can streamline your meal prep process, making it easier to stick to your metabolic diet and reach your health goals.

BREAKFAST RECIPES FOR A METABOLIC BOOST

Energizing Smoothies and Shakes

Incorporating energizing smoothies and shakes into your breakfast routine can provide a metabolic boost to start your day off right. Some recipes are designed to energize your body, support metabolism, and keep you satisfied until your next meal.

Green Metabolism Booster Smoothie

Ingredients:

- 1 cup baby spinach

- 1/2 cup cucumber, chopped

- 1/2 green apple, chopped

- 1/2 avocado

- 1 tablespoon chia seeds

- 1 cup unsweetened almond milk

- A handful of ice cubes

- Juice of 1/2 lemon

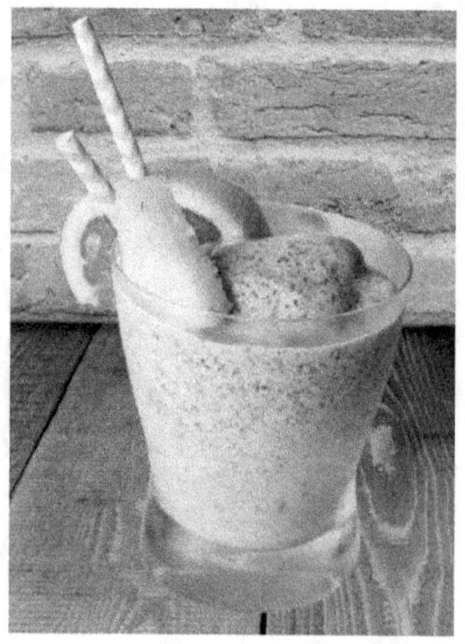

Instructions:

Blend all ingredients until smooth. The combination of fiber from the greens and apple, along with healthy fats from the avocado and chia seeds, kickstarts your metabolism and provides lasting energy.

Berry Protein Power Shake

Ingredients:

- 1 cup mixed berries (strawberries, blueberries, raspberries)

- 1 scoop vanilla or berry-flavored protein powder

- 1 tablespoon ground flaxseed

- 1 cup unsweetened Greek yogurt

- 1/2 cup unsweetened almond milk or water

- A handful of ice cubes

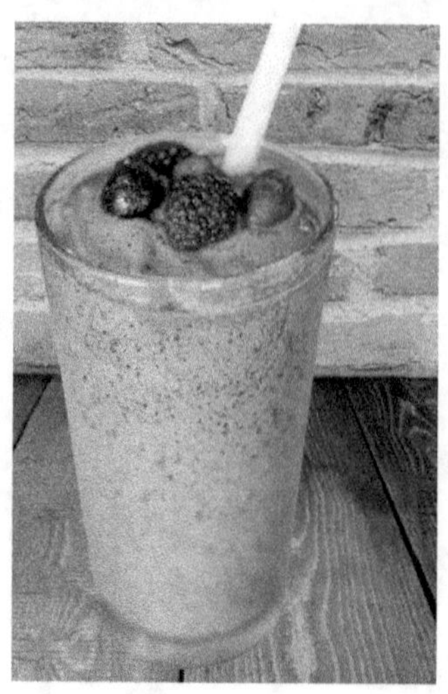

Instructions:

Put all the ingredients in a blender and process until they are smooth. This shake is packed with protein and antioxidants, supporting muscle health and metabolic function.

Tropical Metabolism Kickstart Smoothie

Ingredients:

- 1/2 cup pineapple, chopped

- 1/2 cup mango, chopped

- 1/2 banana

- 1 tablespoon coconut oil

- 1 cup unsweetened coconut milk

- A pinch of cayenne pepper

- A handful of ice cubes

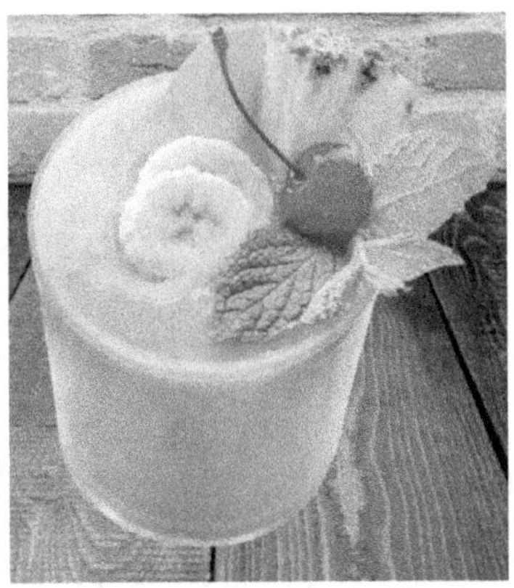

Instructions:

Blend all ingredients until creamy. The medium-chain triglycerides in coconut oil and the capsaicin in cayenne pepper help boost metabolism, while the fruits provide a natural sweetness and energy.

Ingredients:

- 1 banana

- 2 tablespoons almond butter

- 1 tablespoon cocoa powder

- 1 cup unsweetened almond milk

- 1/2 teaspoon cinnamon

- A handful of ice cubes

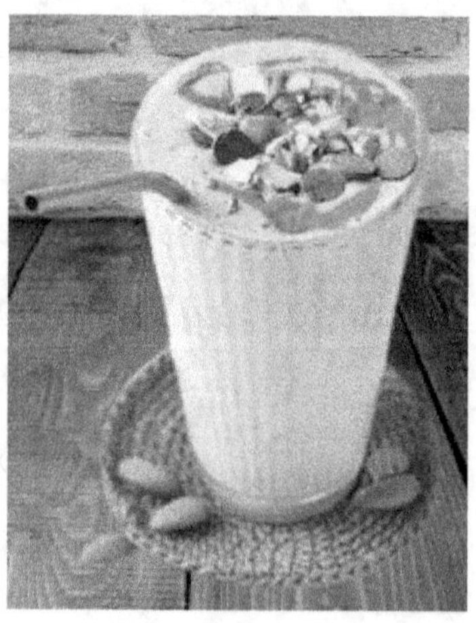

Instructions:

Blend all ingredients until smooth. This smoothie combines the metabolic benefits of cinnamon with the healthy fats in almond butter for a satisfying and energizing start to your day.

Ginger Zing Detox Shake

Ingredients:

- 1 small piece of ginger, peeled and chopped

- 1/2 lemon, juiced

- 1 apple, chopped

- 1 tablespoon honey (optional)

- 1 cup water or green tea, chilled

- A handful of ice cubes

Instructions:

Blend all ingredients until smooth. Ginger and lemon are great for boosting metabolism and detoxifying the body, while the apple and honey add a touch of sweetness.

These smoothies and shakes are not only delicious but also packed with nutrients that support a healthy metabolism. Enjoy these energizing recipes as part of your metabolic diet breakfast routine for a vibrant start to your day.

Protein-Packed Egg Dishes

Eggs are a fantastic source of high-quality protein and other essential nutrients, making them an excellent choice for a metabolism-boosting breakfast. Here are some protein-packed egg dishes that are perfect for a metabolic diet:

Spinach and Feta Egg Muffins

Ingredients:

- 6 large eggs

- 1 cup fresh spinach, chopped

- 1/2 cup feta cheese, crumbled

- 1/4 cup red bell pepper, diced

- Salt and pepper to taste

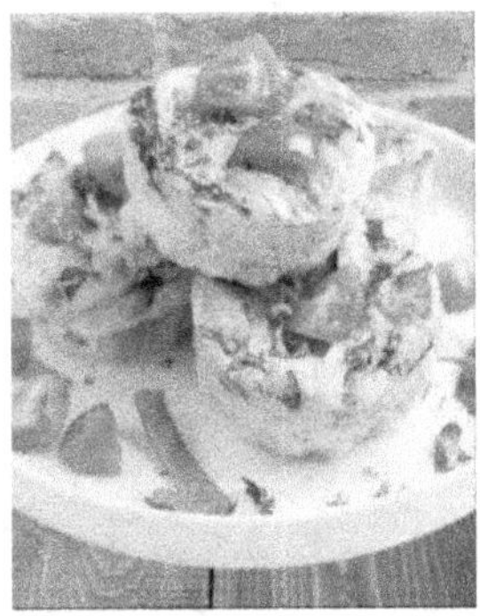

Instructions:

1. Preheat the oven to 350°F (175°C).

2. In a bowl, whisk the eggs. Add the spinach, feta cheese, red bell pepper, salt, and pepper. Mix well.

3. Pour the mixture into greased muffin cups, filling each about 2/3 full.

4. Bake for 20-25 minutes, or until the muffins are set and lightly golden on top.

5. Let cool for a few minutes before serving.

Avocado and Egg Breakfast Bowl

Ingredients:

- 2 large eggs

- 1/2 avocado, sliced

- 1/2 cup cooked quinoa

- 1 cup kale, sautéed

- 1 tablespoon olive oil

- Salt and pepper to taste

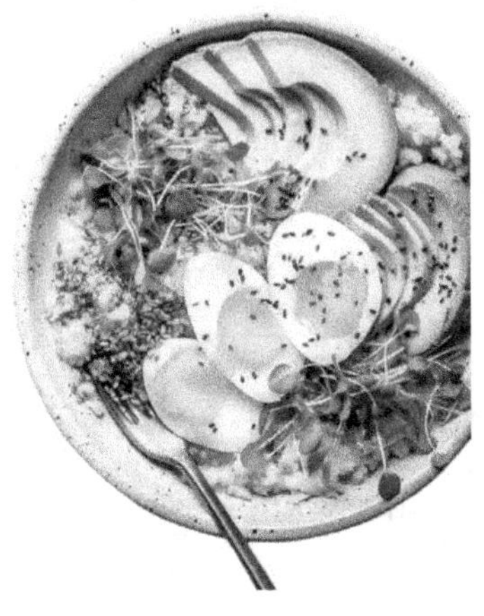

Instructions:

1. Cook the eggs to your preference (boiled, poached, or scrambled).

2. In a bowl, layer the cooked quinoa, sautéed kale, sliced avocado, and cooked eggs.

3. Add a drizzle of olive oil and season with pepper and salt

4. Mix gently and enjoy.

Wholesome Oatmeal and Porridge Variations

Oatmeal and porridge are excellent breakfast options for a metabolic boost, as they are rich in fiber, which helps regulate blood sugar levels and keeps you feeling full longer. Here are some wholesome variations to start your day:

Apple Cinnamon Oatmeal

Ingredients:

- 1 cup rolled oats

- 2 cups water or milk (almond, oat, or cow's)

- 1 apple, diced

- 1 teaspoon ground cinnamon

- 1 tablespoon maple syrup or honey

- A pinch of salt

Instructions:

1. In a pot, put water or milk in a boil.

2. Add oats, diced apple, cinnamon, and salt. Reduce heat and simmer for 5-7 minutes, stirring occasionally.

3. Serve with a drizzle of maple syrup or honey.

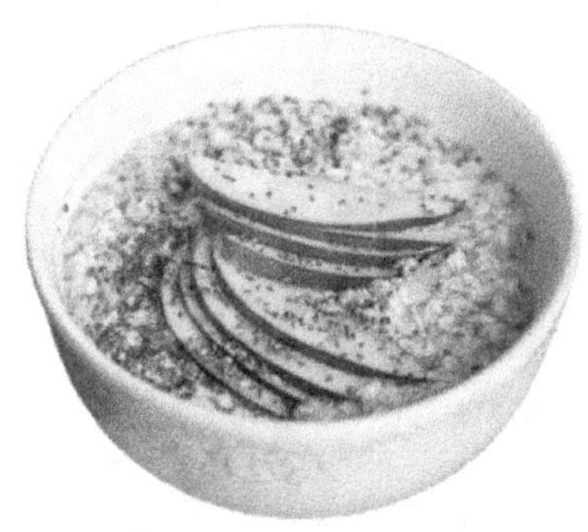

Berry Almond Overnight Oats

Ingredients:

- 1/2 cup rolled oats

- 1/2 cup Greek yogurt

- 2/3 cup almond milk

- 1 tablespoon chia seeds

- 1/2 cup mixed berries (fresh or frozen)

- 1 tablespoon sliced almonds

- 1 tablespoon honey or maple syrup

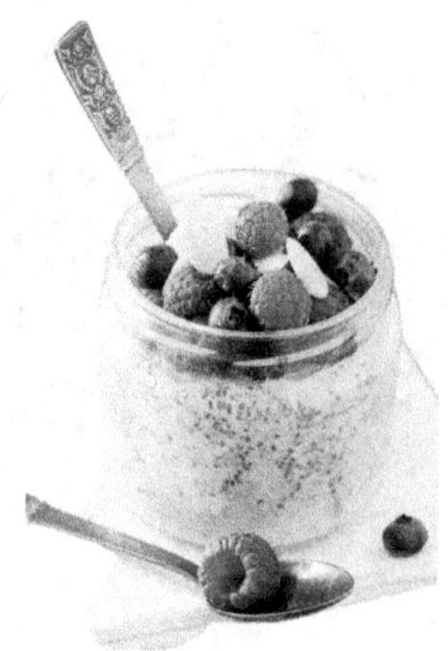

Instructions:

1. In a jar, combine oats, Greek yogurt, almond milk, chia seeds, and honey or maple syrup.

2. Top with mixed berries and sliced almonds.

3. Seal the jar and refrigerate overnight. Stir before eating.

Banana Nut Porridge

Ingredients:

- 1/2 cup quinoa or millet

- 1 cup water

- 1 ripe banana, mashed

- 1/4 cup chopped walnuts

- 1/2 teaspoon vanilla extract

- 1/4 teaspoon ground cinnamon

- Milk or almond milk, for serving

Instructions:

1. Rinse quinoa or millet and add to a pot with water. After bringing to a boil, lower the heat and simmer for 15 minutes with a lid on..

2. Stir in mashed banana, walnuts, vanilla, and cinnamon. Cook for an additional 5 minutes.

3. Serve with a splash of milk or almond milk.

Pumpkin Spice Oatmeal

Ingredients:

- 1 cup rolled oats

- 2 cups water or milk

- 1/2 cup pumpkin puree

- 1 teaspoon pumpkin pie spice

- 1 tablespoon maple syrup or honey

- A pinch of salt

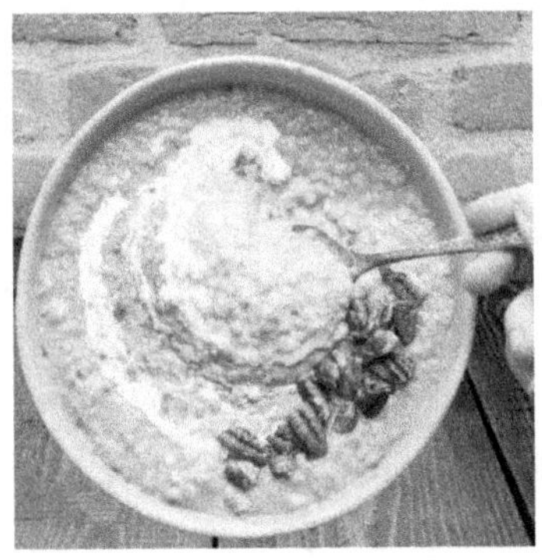

Instructions:

Heat up some water in a saucepan.

Add oats, pumpkin puree, pumpkin pie spice, and salt. Reduce heat and simmer for 5-7 minutes, stirring occasionally.

Serve with a drizzle of maple syrup or honey.

Savory Mushroom and Spinach Oatmeal

Ingredients:

- 1 cup rolled oats

- 2 cups water or vegetable broth

- 1 cup sliced mushrooms

- 2 cups baby spinach

- 1 tablespoon olive oil

- Salt and pepper to taste

- Grated Parmesan cheese (optional)

Instructions:

1. In a pot, cook oats in water or vegetable broth according to package instructions.

2. Heat the olive oil in a separate pan over medium heat. After adding, sauté the sliced mushrooms until browned.

3. Cook the spinach in the pan until it wilts.

4. Stir the mushroom and spinach mixture into the cooked oatmeal. Season with salt and pepper.

5. Serve with grated Parmesan cheese if desired.

These oatmeal and porridge variations are not only delicious but also packed with nutrients that support a healthy metabolism, making them ideal for a wholesome breakfast.

LUNCH RECIPES TO FUEL YOUR DAY

Nutrient-Dense Salads

Nutrient-dense salads are perfect for lunch, providing a balanced meal that fuels your day with vitamins, minerals, fiber, and healthy fats. Some recipes to keep you energized and satisfied:

Quinoa and Black Bean Salad

Ingredients:

- 1 cup cooked quinoa

- 1 can black beans, drained and rinsed

- 1 cup cherry tomatoes, halved

- 1 avocado, diced

- 1/2 red onion, finely chopped

- 1/4 cup fresh cilantro, chopped

- Juice of 1 lime

- 2 tablespoons olive oil

- Salt and pepper to taste

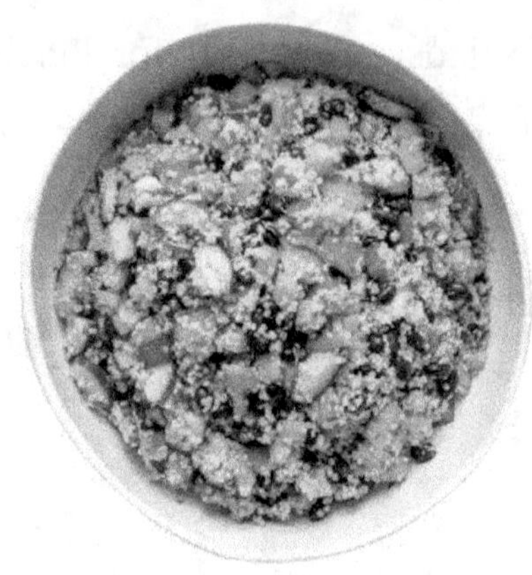

Instructions:

1. In a large bowl, combine quinoa, black beans, cherry tomatoes, avocado, red onion, and cilantro.

2. In a small bowl, whisk together lime juice, olive oil, salt, and pepper.

3. Pour the dressing over the salad and toss to combine. Serve chilled or at room temperature.

Kale and Roasted Sweet Potato Salad

Ingredients:

- 2 cups kale, stems removed and leaves chopped

- 1 large sweet potato, cubed and roasted

- 1/4 cup dried cranberries

- 1/4 cup pecans, toasted

- 2 tablespoons feta cheese, crumbled

- 2 tablespoons balsamic vinaigrette

Instructions:

1. In a large bowl, massage kale with a bit of olive oil until slightly softened.

2. Add roasted sweet potato, dried cranberries, pecans, and feta cheese to the kale.

3. Drizzle with balsamic vinaigrette and toss to combine. Serve immediately.

Ingredients:

- 2 cups shredded cabbage (mix of red and green)

- 1 cup shredded carrots

- 1 cup cooked chicken breast, shredded

- 1/4 cup sliced almonds

- 1/4 cup chopped green onions

- 2 tablespoons sesame seeds

- For the dressing:

- 2 tablespoons soy sauce

- 1 tablespoon rice vinegar

- 1 tablespoon sesame oil

- 1 teaspoon honey

- 1 garlic clove, minced

- 1 teaspoon grated ginger

Instructions:

1. In a large bowl, combine cabbage, carrots, chicken, almonds, green onions, and sesame seeds.

2. In a small bowl, whisk together the dressing ingredients.

3. Pour the dressing over the salad and toss to coat. Serve chilled.

Mediterranean Chickpea Salad

Ingredients:

- 1 can chickpeas, drained and rinsed

- 1 cucumber, diced

- 1 bell pepper, diced

- 1/2 red onion, finely chopped

- 1/4 cup kalamata olives, halved

- 1/4 cup feta cheese, crumbled

- 1/4 cup fresh parsley, chopped

- 2 tablespoons olive oil

- 1 tablespoon lemon juice

- 1 teaspoon dried oregano

- Salt and pepper to taste

Instructions:

1. In a large bowl, combine chickpeas, cucumber, bell pepper, red onion, olives, feta cheese, and parsley.

2. In a small bowl, whisk together olive oil, lemon juice, oregano, salt, and pepper.

3. Pour the dressing over the salad and toss to combine. Serve chilled or at room temperature.

These nutrient-dense salads are not only delicious but also packed with a variety of ingredients that support a healthy metabolism and provide sustained energy throughout the day.

Hearty Soups and Stews

Hearty soups and stews are perfect for a metabolic diet lunch, as they can be packed with protein, fiber, and nutrient-dense vegetables to keep your metabolism humming all day long. Here are some recipes to fuel your day:

Chicken and Vegetable Soup

Ingredients:

- 2 chicken breasts, diced

- 2 carrots, diced

- 2 celery stalks, diced

- 1 onion, chopped

- 2 cloves garlic, minced

- 4 cups low-sodium chicken broth

- 1 cup kale, chopped

- 1 teaspoon dried thyme

- Salt and pepper to taste

Instructions:

1. Sauté onion and garlic in a large pot until translucent.

2. Add chicken and cook until browned.

3. Add carrots, celery, chicken broth, thyme, salt, and pepper. Bring to a boil.

4. Simmer on low heat for 20 minutes.

5. Add kale and cook for an additional 5 minutes. Serve hot.

Beef and Barley Stew

Ingredients:

- 1-pound lean beef stew meat, cubed

- 1 cup barley, rinsed

- 3 carrots, chopped

- 2 parsnips, chopped

- 1 onion, chopped

- 4 cups low-sodium beef broth

- 1 teaspoon dried rosemary

- Salt and pepper to taste

Instructions:

1. Brown beef in a large pot.

2. Add onion and cook until softened.

3. Add beef broth, barley, carrots, parsnips, rosemary, salt, and pepper.

4. Bring to a boil, then reduce heat and simmer for 1 hour, or until barley and vegetables are tender.

Spicy Lentil and Tomato Soup

Ingredients:

- 1 cup lentils, rinsed

- 1 can diced tomatoes

- 1 onion, chopped

- 2 cloves garlic, minced

- 4 cups vegetable broth

- 1 teaspoon cumin

- 1 teaspoon chili powder

- Salt and pepper to taste

Instructions:

1.   Sauté onion and garlic in a large pot until translucent.

2.   Add lentils, diced tomatoes, vegetable broth, cumin, chili powder, salt, and pepper.

3.   Bring to a boil, then reduce heat and simmer for 25-30 minutes, or until lentils are tender.

Turkey and White Bean Chili

Ingredients:

- 1 pound ground turkey

- 1 onion, chopped

- 2 cloves garlic, minced

- One can of washed and drained white beans

- 1 can green chilies

- 4 cups low-sodium chicken broth

- 1 teaspoon ground cumin

- Salt and pepper to taste

Instructions:

1.   Cook ground turkey in a large pot until browned.

2.   Add onion and garlic and cook until softened.

3.   Stir in white beans, green chilies, chicken broth, cumin, salt, and pepper.

4.   4. Boil for four minutes, then lower the heat and simmer for twenty.

Vegetable and Quinoa Soup

Ingredients:

- 1 cup quinoa, rinsed

- 1 carrot, diced

- 1 zucchini, diced

- 1 bell pepper, diced

- 1 onion, chopped

- 4 cups vegetable broth

- 1 teaspoon dried oregano

- Salt and pepper to taste

Instructions:

1. Sauté onion in a large pot until translucent.

2. Add carrot, zucchini, bell pepper, vegetable broth, oregano, salt, and pepper.

3. Bring to a boil, then add quinoa and reduce heat to simmer for 20 minutes, or until quinoa is cooked and vegetables are tender.

These soups and stews are not only delicious and satisfying but also align with the principles of a metabolic diet, providing balanced nutrition to keep your energy levels up throughout the day.

Wraps and Sandwiches with a Metabolic Twist

Wraps and sandwiches are versatile and convenient options for a metabolic diet lunch. By choosing the right ingredients, you can create delicious and nutritious meals that fuel your day and support your metabolism. Here are some recipes with a metabolic twist:

Turkey Avocado Wrap

Ingredients:

- Whole wheat or low-carb wrap

- Sliced turkey breast

- 1/4 avocado, sliced

- Mixed greens (spinach, arugula, etc.)

- Sliced tomato

- Mustard or hummus for spread

Instructions:

1. Lay the wrap flat on a plate.

2. Spread mustard or hummus over the wrap.

   1. Layer turkey, avocado slices, mixed greens, and tomato on the wrap.

   2. Roll up the wrap tightly and cut it in half.

Grilled Chicken and Veggie Pita

Ingredients:

- Whole wheat pita bread

- Grilled chicken breast, sliced

- Roasted bell peppers

- Sliced cucumber

- Mixed greens

- Tzatziki sauce or Greek yogurt

Instructions:

1.   Cut the pita bread in half to form pockets.

2.   Spread tzatziki sauce or Greek yogurt inside each pita half.

3.   Fill with grilled chicken, roasted bell peppers, cucumber, and mixed greens.

Spicy Tuna Salad Wrap

Ingredients:

- Whole wheat or low-carb wrap

- Canned tuna in water, drained

- Greek yogurt (as a mayo substitute)

- Diced celery

- Diced red onion

- A pinch of cayenne pepper

- Sliced lettuce

Instructions:

1. In a bowl, mix tuna, Greek yogurt, celery, red onion, and cayenne pepper.

2. Lay the wrap flat and place lettuce leaves in the center.

3. Add the tuna salad mixture on top of the lettuce.

4. Roll up the wrap tightly and cut in half.

Hummus and Roasted Veggie Sandwich

Ingredients:

- Whole grain bread

- Hummus

- Roasted vegetables (eggplant, zucchini, bell peppers)

- Sliced avocado

- Alfalfa sprouts or micro greens

Instructions:

1. Spread hummus on two slices of whole-grain bread.

2. Layer roasted vegetables, avocado slices, and alfalfa sprouts on one slice of bread.

3. Top with the other slice of bread and cut the sandwich in half.

- Hearty Soups and Stews

- Wraps and Sandwiches with a Metabolic Twist

Ingredients:

- Whole-grain bread

- Sliced turkey breast

- Thinly sliced apple

- Brie cheese

- Baby spinach

- Dijon mustard

Instructions:

1. Spread Dijon mustard on two slices of whole-grain bread.

2. Layer turkey, apple slices, Brie, and baby spinach on one slice of bread.

3. Top with the other slice of bread and grill in a panini press or on a skillet until the cheese is melted and the bread is toasted.

These wraps and sandwiches provide a balance of lean proteins, healthy fats, fiber, and complex carbohydrates, all of which contribute to a well-functioning metabolism. Enjoy these recipes for a satisfying and energizing lunch!

DINNER RECIPES FOR METABOLIC SUPPORT

Lean Protein Entrees

Lean protein is a crucial component of a metabolic diet, as it helps build muscle, boost metabolism, and keep you feeling full. Here are some dinner recipes featuring lean protein that are perfect for a metabolic diet:

Grilled Lemon Herb Chicken

Ingredients:

- 4 boneless, skinless chicken breasts

- Juice of 1 lemon

- 2 cloves garlic, minced

- 1 tablespoon olive oil

- 1 teaspoon dried oregano

- Salt and pepper to taste

Instructions:

1. In a bowl, mix lemon juice, garlic, olive oil, oregano, salt, and pepper.

2. For a minimum of half an hour, marinate chicken breasts in the marinade.

3. Preheat the grill to medium-high heat and grill chicken for 6-7 minutes per side, or until cooked through.

Baked Salmon with Dill Yogurt Sauce

Ingredients:

- 4 salmon fillets

- 1 cup Greek yogurt

- 2 tablespoons chopped fresh dill

- 1 tablespoon lemon juice

- 1 clove garlic, minced

- Salt and pepper to taste

Instructions:

1. Preheat oven to 400°F (200°C).

2. Season salmon fillets with salt and pepper and place on a baking sheet.

3. Bake for 12-15 minutes, or until salmon flakes easily with a fork.

4. In a small bowl, mix Greek yogurt, dill, lemon juice, garlic, salt, and pepper.

5. Serve salmon with a dollop of dill yogurt sauce on top.

Turkey and Quinoa Stuffed Peppers

Ingredients:

- 4 bell peppers, halved and seeded

- 1-pound lean ground turkey

- 1 cup cooked quinoa

- 1 can diced tomatoes, drained

- 1 onion, chopped

- 2 cloves garlic, minced

- 1 teaspoon cumin

- 1 teaspoon smoked paprika

- Salt and pepper to taste

- Shredded cheese (optional)

Instructions:

1. Preheat oven to 375°F (190°C).

2. In a skillet, cook ground turkey, onion, and garlic until turkey is browned.

3. Stir in quinoa, diced tomatoes, cumin, smoked paprika, salt, and pepper.

4. Fill each bell pepper half with the turkey and quinoa mixture.

5. Place stuffed peppers in a baking dish and bake for 25-30 minutes.

6. Top with shredded cheese in the last 5 minutes of baking if desired.

Grilled Shrimp and Vegetable Skewers

Ingredients:

- 1 pound of big, peeled and deveined shrimp

- 2 zucchinis, sliced

- 2 bell peppers, cut into chunks

- 1 red onion, cut into chunks

- 2 tablespoons olive oil

- 1 tablespoon lemon juice

- 2 cloves garlic, minced

- Salt and pepper to taste

Instructions:

1. In a bowl, mix olive oil, lemon juice, garlic, salt, and pepper.

2. Thread shrimp, zucchini, bell peppers, and red onion onto skewers.

3. Brush skewers with the olive oil mixture.

4. Preheat grill to medium-high heat and grill skewers for 2-3 minutes per side, or until shrimp is cooked through.

Lemon Garlic Tilapia

Ingredients:

- 4 tilapia fillets

- Juice of 1 lemon

- 2 cloves garlic, minced

- 2 tablespoons olive oil

- 1 teaspoon dried parsley

- Salt and pepper to taste

Instructions:

1. Preheat oven to 400°F (200°C).

2. In a small bowl, mix lemon juice, garlic, olive oil, parsley, salt, and pepper.

3. Place tilapia fillets in a baking dish and pour the lemon garlic mixture over them.

4. Bake for 10-12 minutes, or until fish flakes easily with a fork.

These lean protein entrees are not only delicious but also support a healthy metabolism, making them ideal for a metabolic diet dinner.

Vegetarian and Vegan

Incorporating vegetarian and vegan options into a metabolic diet can be both delicious and nutritious. Here are some dinner recipes that are perfect for those following a plant-based metabolic diet:

Chickpea and Sweet Potato Curry

Ingredients:

- 1 tablespoon coconut oil

- 1 onion, diced

- 2 cloves garlic, minced

- 1 tablespoon grated ginger

- 1 tablespoon curry powder

- 1 can chickpeas, drained and rinsed

- 1 large sweet potato, peeled and cubed

- 1 can of coconut milk

- Salt and pepper to taste

- Fresh cilantro for garnish

Instructions:

1. In a large saucepan set over medium heat, warm the coconut oil.

2. Sauté onion, garlic, and ginger until softened.

3. Add curry powder and cook for 1 minute.

4. Add chickpeas, sweet potato, and coconut milk. Season with salt and pepper.

5. Bring to a boil, then reduce heat and simmer for 20 minutes, or until sweet potatoes are tender.

Ingredients:

- 4 bell peppers, cut in half, and seeds taken out

- 1 cup cooked quinoa

- 1 can black beans, drained and rinsed

- 1 cup corn kernels

- 1 teaspoon cumin

- 1 teaspoon chili powder

- Salt and pepper to taste

- Shredded vegan cheese (optional)

Instructions:

1. Preheat oven to 375°F (190°C).

2. In a bowl, mix quinoa, black beans, corn, cumin, chili powder, salt, and pepper.

3. Fill each bell pepper half with the quinoa mixture.

4. Place stuffed peppers in a baking dish and bake for 25-30 minutes.

5. Top with shredded vegan cheese in the last 5 minutes of baking if desired.

Lentil and Mushroom Bolognese

Ingredients:

- 1 tablespoon olive oil

- 1 onion, diced

- 2 cloves garlic, minced

- 1 cup brown lentils, rinsed

- 2 cups vegetable broth

- 1 can crushed tomatoes

- 1 cup chopped mushrooms

- 1 teaspoon dried oregano

- Salt and pepper to taste

- Cooked whole wheat pasta or zucchini noodles

Instructions:

1. In a large saucepan, bring the olive oil to a temperature of medium.

2. Sauté onion and garlic until softened.

3. Add lentils, vegetable broth, crushed tomatoes, mushrooms, oregano, salt, and pepper.

4. After bringing to a boil, lower the heat, and simmer the lentils for 25 to 30 minutes, or until they are tender.

5. Serve the Bolognese sauce over cooked pasta or zucchini noodles.

Roasted Cauliflower Steaks with Tahini Sauce

Ingredients:

- 1 large cauliflower, sliced into steaks

- 2 tablespoons olive oil

- Salt and pepper to taste

- 1/4 cup tahini

- 2 tablespoons lemon juice

- 1 clove garlic, minced

- 2-3 tablespoons water

Instructions:

1. Preheat oven to 400°F (200°C).

2. Brush cauliflower steaks with olive oil and season with salt and pepper.

3. Roast in the oven for 25-30 minutes, or until golden and tender.

4. In a small bowl, whisk together tahini, lemon juice, garlic, and water until smooth.

5. Drizzle tahini sauce over roasted cauliflower steaks before serving.

Spinach and Tofu Stir-Fry

Ingredients:

- 1 block of firm tofu, pressed and cubed

- 2 tablespoons soy sauce

- 1 tablespoon sesame oil

- 2 cloves garlic, minced

- 1 teaspoon grated ginger

- 4 cups fresh spinach

- 1 tablespoon sesame seeds

Instructions:

1. Marinate tofu cubes in soy sauce for 15 minutes.

2. Heat sesame oil in a large pan over medium heat.

3. Add garlic and ginger, and sauté for 1 minute.

4. Add tofu and cook until golden brown.

5. Add spinach and cook until wilted.

6. Sprinkle sesame seeds over the stir-fry before serving.

These vegetarian and vegan options are not only delicious but also packed with nutrients that support a healthy metabolism, making them ideal for a metabolic diet dinner.

Satisfying Stir-Fries and Skillet Meals

Stir-fries and skillet meals are excellent options for a metabolic diet dinner, as they can be quickly prepared with a variety of nutrient-dense ingredients. Here are some recipes that are both satisfying and supportive of a healthy metabolism:

Spicy Chicken and Broccoli Stir-Fry

Ingredients:

- 1 pound chicken breast, thinly sliced

- 2 cups broccoli florets

- 1 bell pepper, sliced

- 2 tablespoons olive oil

- 2 cloves garlic, minced

- 1 tablespoon grated ginger

- 2 tablespoons low-sodium soy sauce

- 1 tablespoon chili sauce or sriracha

- Salt and pepper to taste

Instructions:

Within a large skillet, bring the olive oil to a temperature of medium-high.

Add chicken and cook until browned. Remove from skillet and set aside.

In the same skillet, add garlic, ginger, broccoli, and bell pepper. Stir-fry for 3-4 minutes.

Return the chicken to the skillet, add soy sauce and chili sauce, and stir well.

Cook for an additional 2-3 minutes, or until vegetables are tender and chicken is cooked through. Season with salt and pepper.

Tofu and Vegetable Quinoa Stir-Fry

Ingredients:

- 1 block firm tofu, pressed and cubed

- 2 cups cooked quinoa

- 1 cup snap peas

- 1 carrot, sliced

- 1 bell pepper, sliced

- 2 tablespoons coconut oil

- 2 tablespoons tamari or soy sauce

- 1 tablespoon sesame oil

- 1 teaspoon chili flakes (optional)

Instructions:

1.   Heat coconut oil in a large skillet over medium-high heat.

2.   Add tofu and cook until golden brown on all sides.

3. Add snap peas, carrots, and bell pepper to the skillet. Stir-fry for 4-5 minutes.

4. Add cooked quinoa, tamari, sesame oil, and chili flakes. Stir well to combine.

5. Cook for an additional 2-3 minutes, or until vegetables are tender and tofu is heated through.

Beef and Asparagus Skillet

Ingredients:

- 1-pound lean beef, thinly sliced

- 2 cups asparagus, trimmed and cut into pieces

- 1 onion, sliced

- 2 tablespoons olive oil

- 2 cloves garlic, minced

- 2 tablespoons balsamic vinegar

- Salt and pepper to taste

Instructions:

1. Within a large skillet, bring the olive oil to a temperature of medium-high.

2. Add beef and cook until browned. Remove from skillet and set aside.

3. In the same skillet, add onion and garlic. Sauté for 2 minutes.

4. The asparagus should be cooked for three to four minutes, or until it is crisp-tender.

5. Return the beef to the skillet, add balsamic vinegar, and season with salt and pepper. Stir well and cook for more than 2 minutes.

Shrimp and Cauliflower Rice Stir-Fry

Ingredients:

- 1 pound shrimp, peeled and deveined

- 4 cups cauliflower rice

- 1 cup bell pepper, diced

- 1 cup snow peas

- 2 tablespoons olive oil

- 2 cloves garlic, minced

- 2 tablespoons low-sodium soy sauce

- 1 tablespoon lemon juice

Instructions:

1.   Within a large skillet, bring the olive oil to a temperature of medium-high.

2.   Add garlic and shrimp. Cook till shrimp are pink and opaque

3.   Add cauliflower rice, bell pepper, and snow peas. Stir-fry for 5-6 minutes.

4.   Add soy sauce and lemon juice. Mix well and cook for another 2 minutes.

These stir-fries and skillet meals are not only quick and easy to prepare but also packed with lean proteins, vegetables, and healthy fats that support a metabolic diet, making them ideal for a nutritious and satisfying dinner.

Spicy Turkey and Green Bean Skillet

Ingredients:

- 1-pound lean ground turkey

- 2 cups green beans, trimmed and cut into pieces

- 1 onion, diced

- 2 cloves garlic, minced

- 2 tablespoons olive oil

- 1 tablespoon chili powder

- 1 teaspoon cumin

- Salt and pepper to taste

- Fresh cilantro for garnish

Instructions:

1.   Within a large skillet, bring the olive oil to a temperature of medium-high.

2.   Add onion and garlic, sautéing until softened.

3.   Add ground turkey, breaking it apart with a spatula then Cook until browned.

4.   Stir in green beans, chili powder, cumin, salt, and pepper. Cook for 5-7 minutes, or until green beans are tender.

5.   Garnish with fresh cilantro before serving.

Lemon Garlic Salmon and Zucchini Noodles

Ingredients:

- 4 salmon fillets

- 4 cups zucchini noodles (zoodles)

- 2 tablespoons olive oil

- 2 cloves garlic, minced

- Juice and zest of 1 lemon

- Salt and pepper to taste

- Fresh parsley for garnish

Instructions:

1.   Preheat oven to 400°F (200°C).

2.   Place salmon fillets on a baking sheet. Drizzle with olive oil, lemon juice, and zest. Season with salt, pepper, and minced garlic.

3.   Fish should be baked for 12 to 15 minutes, or until it is completely cooked through.

4.   While salmon is baking, heat a separate skillet over medium heat. Add zucchini noodles and sauté for 2-3 minutes, or until slightly softened.

5.   Serve salmon over a bed of zucchini noodles, garnished with fresh parsley.

Chicken and Cauliflower Fried "Rice"

Ingredients:

- 1 pound chicken breast, diced

- 4 cups cauliflower rice

- 1 cup frozen peas and carrots

- 1 onion, diced

- 2 cloves garlic, minced

- 2 tablespoons sesame oil

- 2-3 tablespoons low-sodium soy sauce

- 2 eggs, beaten

- Green onions for garnish

Instructions:

1.	Heat sesame oil in a large skillet or wok over medium-high heat.

2.	Add onion, garlic, and diced chicken. Cook until chicken is browned.

3.	Place the chicken on one side of the skillet, and then add the eggs that have been beaten on the other side. Scramble eggs until cooked.

4.	Add cauliflower rice, peas carrots, and soy sauce. Stir everything together and cook for 5-7 minutes, or until cauliflower rice is tender.

5.	Just before serving, garnish with green onions that have been chopped.

Spicy Black Bean and Quinoa Skillet

Ingredients:

- 1 cup quinoa, cooked

- 1 can black beans, drained and rinsed

- 1 bell pepper, diced

- 1 onion, diced

- 2 cloves garlic, minced

- 2 tablespoons olive oil

- 1 teaspoon chili powder

- 1 teaspoon cumin

- Salt and pepper to taste

- Fresh cilantro for garnish

Instructions:

1.   Within a large skillet, bring the olive oil to a temperature of medium-high.

2.   Add onion, bell pepper, and garlic. Sauté until softened.

3.   Stir in black beans, cooked quinoa, chili powder, cumin, salt, and pepper. Cook for five to seven minutes, or until the food is totally warm.

4.   Garnish with fresh cilantro before serving.

These recipes are not only flavorful and satisfying but also packed with nutrients that support a healthy metabolism, making them ideal choices for a metabolic diet dinner.

SNACKS AND SIDES TO KEEP METABOLISM HUMMING

Crunchy Veggie Snacks

Crunchy veggie snacks are a great way to keep your metabolism humming throughout the day. They provide essential nutrients, fiber, and hydration while satisfying your craving for something crunchy. Here are some ideas for crunchy veggie snacks:

Kale Chips

Ingredients:

- 1 bunch kale, washed and dried
- 1 tablespoon olive oil
- Salt and pepper to taste

Instructions:

1. Preheat oven to 300°F (150°C).

2.   Remove the kale leaves from the stems and tear them into bite-sized pieces.

3.   Toss kale leaves with olive oil, salt, and pepper.

4.   Spread the kale leaves in a single layer on a baking sheet.

5.   Bake for 10-15 minutes, or until crispy. Let cool before serving.

Carrot and Cucumber Sticks with Hummus

Ingredients:

- Carrots, peeled and cut into sticks

- Cucumbers, sliced into sticks

- Hummus for dipping

Instructions:

1.   Prepare carrot and cucumber sticks.

2.   Serve with a side of hummus for dipping.

Bell Pepper Nachos

Ingredients:

- Bell peppers, sliced into rounds

- Shredded cheese (optional)

- Sliced black olives

- Diced tomatoes

- Greek yogurt or sour cream

- Salsa

Instructions:

1.   Preheat oven to 375°F (190°C).

2.   Arrange bell pepper rounds on a baking sheet.

3.   Top with shredded cheese, black olives, and diced tomatoes.

4.   Bake for 5-7 minutes, or until cheese is melted.

5.   Serve with a dollop of Greek yogurt or sour cream and salsa.

Roasted Chickpeas

Ingredients:

- 1 can chickpeas, drained and rinsed

- 1 tablespoon olive oil

- Seasonings of choice (e.g., garlic powder, paprika, cumin)

- Salt to taste

Instructions:

1.   Preheat oven to 400°F (200°C).

2.   Pat chickpeas dry with a towel.

3.   Toss chickpeas with olive oil, seasonings, and salt.

4.   Spread chickpeas on a baking sheet in a single layer.

5.   Roast for 20-30 minutes, shaking the pan halfway through, until crispy.

Jicama Sticks with Lime and Chili Powder

Ingredients:

- 1 jicama, peeled and cut into sticks

- Lime wedges

- Chili powder

- Salt

Instructions:

1.   Arrange jicama sticks on a plate.

2.   Squeeze lime juice over the jicama sticks.

3.   Sprinkle with chili powder and salt to taste.

These crunchy veggie snacks are not only delicious but also provide a healthy boost to your metabolism, making them perfect for snacking or as a side dish.

Nutrient-Dense Salads

Nutrient-dense salads are perfect for lunch, providing a balanced meal that fuels your day with vitamins, minerals, fiber, and healthy fats. Here are some recipes to keep you energized and satisfied:

Quinoa and Black Bean Salad

Ingredients:

- 1 cup of cooked quinoa

- 1 can black beans, drained and rinsed

- 1 cup cherry tomatoes, halved

- 1 avocado, diced

- 1/2 red onion, finely chopped

- 1/4 cup fresh cilantro, chopped

- Juice of 1 lime

- 2 tablespoons of olive oil

- Salt and pepper to taste

Instructions:

1. In a large bowl, combine quinoa, black beans, cherry tomatoes, avocado, red onion, and cilantro.

2. In a small bowl, combine the lime juice, olive oil, salt, and pepper by carefully whisking them together.

After pouring the dressing over the salad, toss it to incorporate the ingredients. Serve chilled or at room temperature.

Ingredients:

- 2 cups kale, stems removed, and leaves chopped

- 1 large sweet potato, cubed and roasted

- 1/4 cup dried cranberries

- 1/4 cup pecans, toasted

- 2 tablespoons feta cheese, crumbled

- 2 tablespoons balsamic vinaigrette

Instructions:

1. In a large bowl, massage kale with a bit of olive oil until slightly softened.

2. Add roasted sweet potatoes, dried cranberries, pecans, and feta cheese to the kale.

3. Drizzle with balsamic vinaigrette and toss to combine. Serve immediately.

Asian Chicken and Cabbage Salad

Ingredients:

- 2 cups shredded cabbage (mix of red and green)

- 1 cup shredded carrots

- 1 cup cooked chicken breast, shredded

- 1/4 cup sliced almonds

- 1/4 cup chopped green onions

- 2 tablespoons of sesame seeds

- For the dressing:

- 2 tablespoons of soy sauce

- 1 tablespoon of rice vinegar

- 1 tablespoon sesame oil

- 1 teaspoon of honey

- 1 garlic clove, minced

- 1 teaspoon grated ginger

Instructions:

1. In a large bowl, combine the cabbage, carrots, chicken, almonds, green onions, and sesame seeds.

2. In a small bowl, combine the lime juice, olive oil, salt, and pepper by carefully whisking them together.

3. After pouring the dressing over the salad, toss it to incorporate the ingredients. Serve chilled.

Mediterranean Chickpea Salad

Ingredients:

- 1 can chickpeas, drained and rinsed

- 1 cucumber, diced

- 1 bell pepper, diced

- 1/2 red onion, finely chopped

- 1/4 cup kalamata olives, halved

- 1/4 cup feta cheese, crumbled

- 1/4 cup fresh parsley, chopped

- 2 tablespoons of olive oil

- 1 tablespoon of lemon juice

- 1 teaspoon dried oregano

- Salt and pepper to taste

Instructions:

1. Place the chickpeas, cucumber, bell pepper, red onion, olives, feta cheese, and parsley in a large bowl and mix everything.

2. Place the olive oil, lemon juice, oregano, salt, and pepper in a small bowl and mix all of the ingredients.

3. Cover the salad with the dressing and toss it to mix the ingredients. Serve chilled or at room temperature.

These nutrient-dense salads are not only delicious but also packed with a variety of ingredients that support a healthy metabolism and provide sustained energy throughout the day.

Healthy Baked Goods Snacks

Healthy baked goods can be a great way to satisfy your snack cravings while keeping your metabolism humming. Here are some recipes for snacks and sides that are nutritious and delicious:

Ingredients:

- 1 1/2 cups whole wheat flour

- 1 teaspoon baking soda

- 1/2 teaspoon baking powder

- 1 teaspoon cinnamon

- 1/2 teaspoon nutmeg

- 1/4 teaspoon salt

- 1/2 cup unsweetened applesauce

- 1/4 cup honey or maple syrup

- 2 eggs

- 1 teaspoon of vanilla extract

- 1 1/2 cups grated zucchini

- 1/2 cup chopped walnuts (optional)

Instructions:

1. Preheat the oven to 350°F (175°C). Paper liners should be used to line a muffin tray.

2. Combine the flour, baking soda, baking powder, cinnamon, nutmeg, and salt in a bowl and mix them utilizing a whisk.

3. mix applesauce, honey, eggs, and vanilla in another bowl. Stir in grated zucchini.

4. You should mix the dry components with the liquid ingredients until they are almost completely incorporated. Fold in walnuts if using.

5. Divide the batter into muffin cups and bake for 20–25 minutes, or until a toothpick comes out clean.

Oatmeal Banana Breakfast Cookies

Ingredients:

- 2 ripe bananas, mashed

- 1 1/2 cups rolled oats

- 1/2 cup almond butter or peanut butter

- 1/4 cup chopped nuts or seeds

- 1/4 cup dried fruit (raisins, cranberries, etc.)

- 1 teaspoon cinnamon

- 1 teaspoon of vanilla extract

Instructions:

1. Preheat the oven to 350°F (175°C). Place parchment paper on a baking pan and set it aside.

2. In a bowl, mix mashed bananas, oats, almond butter, nuts, dried fruit, cinnamon, and vanilla.

3. Drop spoonful of the mixture onto the baking sheet and flatten slightly.

4. Bake for 12–15 minutes, or until the edges are golden. Let it cool before serving.

Pumpkin Spice Energy Bars

Ingredients:

- 1 cup dates, pitted

- 1 cup rolled oats

- 1/2 cup pumpkin puree

- 1/4 cup almonds

- 1/4 cup pumpkin seeds

- 2 teaspoons of pumpkin pie spice

- 1 teaspoon of vanilla extract

- Pinch of salt

Instructions:

1. In a food processor, blend dates, oats, pumpkin puree, almonds, pumpkin seeds, pumpkin pie spice, vanilla, and salt until well combined.

2. Press the mixture into a lined square baking dish.

3. Refrigerate for at least 2 hours, then cut into bars.

Sweet Potato and Black Bean Quesadillas (baked)

Ingredients:

- 1 medium sweet potato, cooked and mashed

- 1 can black beans, drained and rinsed

- 1/2 teaspoon cumin

- 1/4 teaspoon chili powder

- Whole wheat tortillas

- 1/2 cup shredded cheese (optional)

Instructions:

1. Preheat the oven to 400°F (200°C).

2. Mix mashed sweet potatoes, black beans, cumin, and chili powder.

3. Spread the mixture onto half of each tortilla, sprinkle with cheese if using, and fold over.

4. Place quesadillas on a baking sheet and bake for 10–15 minutes, flipping halfway, until crispy.

These healthy baked goods are perfect for keeping your metabolism active and providing you with sustained energy throughout the day. Enjoy them as snacks or sides to complement your meals!

Whole-Grain Sides

Whole-grain sides are an excellent addition to your snacks and meals, providing essential nutrients, fiber, and energy to keep your metabolism humming. Here are some recipes for whole-grain snacks and sides that are both nutritious and delicious:

Quinoa Tabouleh

Ingredients:

- 1 cup of cooked quinoa

- 1 cup chopped, fresh parsley

- 1/2 cup chopped fresh mint

- 2 tomatoes, diced

- 1 cucumber, diced

- 3 green onions, thinly sliced

- 1/4 cup of lemon juice

- 2 tablespoons of olive oil

- Salt and pepper to taste

Instructions:

1. combine quinoa, parsley, mint, tomatoes, cucumber, and green onions in a large bowl.

2. Place the lemon juice, olive oil, salt, and pepper in a small bowl and mix all of the ingredients together.

3. After pouring the dressing over the quinoa mixture, toss it to blend the ingredients.

Whole Wheat Pita Chips

Ingredients:

- Whole wheat pita bread

- Olive oil

- Garlic powder

- Paprika

- Salt

Instructions:

1. Preheat the oven to 375°F (190°C).

2. Cut pita bread into triangles and arrange on a baking sheet.

3. Lightly brush each pita triangle with olive oil.

4. Sprinkle with garlic powder, paprika, and salt.

5. Bake for 10–12 minutes, or until crispy and golden. Let it cool before serving.

Brown Rice and Vegetable Stir-Fry

Ingredients:

- 1 cup of cooked brown rice

- 1 tablespoon of olive oil

- 2 cups mixed vegetables (bell peppers, carrots, broccoli, and peas)

- 2 cloves garlic, minced

- 2 tablespoons soy sauce or tamari

- 1 teaspoon sesame oil

- 1 teaspoon grated ginger

Instructions:

1. In a large skillet or wok, bring the olive oil to a temperature on the medium-high side.

2. Add mixed vegetables and garlic, and stir-fry for 5-7 minutes, or until vegetables are tender-crisp.

3. Add cooked brown rice, soy sauce, sesame oil, and ginger. Stir-fry for an additional 2–3 minutes.

4. Serve as a side dish or add a protein of your choice for a complete meal.

Ingredients:

- 1 cup cooked farro

- 2 cups mixed vegetables (zucchini, bell peppers, cherry tomatoes), roasted

- 1/4 cup crumbled feta cheese

- 1/4 cup chopped fresh basil

- 2 tablespoons of balsamic vinegar

- 2 tablespoons of olive oil

- Salt and pepper to taste

Instructions:

1. In a large bowl, combine cooked farro, roasted vegetables, feta cheese, and basil.

2. In a small bowl, whisk together the balsamic vinegar, olive oil, salt, and pepper.

3. Pour the dressing over the farro mixture and toss to combine. Serve at room temperature or chilled.

These whole-grain sides are not only delicious but also packed with nutrients that support a healthy metabolism, making them ideal for snacks or as accompaniments to your main meals.

DESSERTS AND TREATS FOR GUILT-FREE INDULGENCE

Low-Sugar Sweet Treats Desserts and Treats

Indulging in low-sugar sweet treats can satisfy your cravings without derailing your metabolic diet. Here are some recipes for desserts and treats that are guilt-free and delicious:

Avocado Chocolate Mousse

Ingredients:

- 2 ripe avocados

- 1/4 cup unsweetened cocoa powder

- 1/4 cup almond milk

- 2-3 tablespoons maple syrup or honey (adjust to taste)

- 1 teaspoon vanilla extract

- Pinch of salt

Instructions:

Scoop the avocado flesh into a blender or food processor.

Add cocoa powder, almond milk, maple syrup or honey, vanilla extract, and a pinch of salt.

Blend until smooth and creamy.

Before serving, allow the dish to chill in the refrigerator for at least half an hour.

Almond and Coconut Energy Balls

Ingredients:

- 1 cup almonds

- 1 cup dates, pitted

- 1/2 cup shredded unsweetened coconut

- 1 tablespoon chia seeds

* 1 tablespoon coconut oil

* 1 teaspoon vanilla extract

Instructions:

In a food processor, blend almonds until finely ground.

Add dates, shredded coconut, chia seeds, coconut oil, and vanilla extract. Blend until the mixture comes together.

Roll the mixture into small balls and refrigerate for at least 30 minutes before serving.

Baked Apple Chips

Ingredients:

* 2-3 apples, thinly sliced

* Cinnamon (optional)

Instructions:

Preheat oven to 200°F (95°C).

Arrange apple slices in a single layer on a baking sheet lined with parchment paper.

Sprinkle with cinnamon if desired.

Bake for 2-3 hours, flipping halfway through, until the apple slices are dried and crispy.

Greek Yogurt and Berry Parfaits

Ingredients:

- 2 cups Greek yogurt

- 1 cup mixed berries (strawberries, blueberries, raspberries)

- 1/4 cup granola (optional)

- Honey or maple syrup (optional)

Instructions:

In serving glasses, layer Greek yogurt, berries, and granola.

Drizzle with a little honey or maple syrup if desired.

Repeat the layers until the glasses are filled.

Peanut Butter and Banana Ice Cream

Ingredients:

- 3 ripe bananas, sliced and frozen

- 2 tablespoons natural peanut butter

- 1 teaspoon vanilla extract

Instructions:

1.   Place frozen banana slices in a food processor or high-speed blender.

2.   Add peanut butter and vanilla extract.

3.   Blend until smooth and creamy, resembling soft-serve ice cream.

4.   Serve immediately or freeze for a firmer texture.

These low-sugar sweet treats are perfect for satisfying your sweet tooth while keeping your metabolism in check. Enjoy them as a guilt-free indulgence anytime!

Fruit-Based Desserts and Treats

Fruit-based desserts are a wonderful way to satisfy your sweet tooth while keeping things healthy and guilt-free. Here are some delicious recipes that celebrate the natural sweetness of fruits:

Grilled Peaches with Honey and Yogurt

Ingredients:

- 4 ripe peaches, halved and pitted

- 1 tablespoon olive oil

- 1 cup Greek yogurt

- 2 tablespoons honey

- A pinch of cinnamon (optional)

Instructions:

1. Preheat your grill to medium heat.

2. Brush the cut sides of the peaches with olive oil.

3. Place the peaches cut-side down on the grill and cook for 4-5 minutes, or until grill marks appear.

4. Serve the grilled peaches with a dollop of Greek yogurt, a drizzle of honey, and a sprinkle of cinnamon.

Berry and Kiwi Fruit Salad

Ingredients:

- 1 cup strawberries, sliced

- 1 cup blueberries

- 2 kiwis, peeled and sliced

- 1 tablespoon fresh mint, chopped

- 1 tablespoon lime juice

- 1 teaspoon honey (optional)

Instructions:

1.   In a large bowl, combine the strawberries, blueberries, and kiwis.

2.   In a small bowl, mix lime juice, honey, and chopped mint.

3.   Pour the dressing over the fruit salad and gently toss to combine.

Ingredients:

- 4 apples, cored

- 1/4 cup chopped walnuts or pecans

- 2 tablespoons raisins

- 1 teaspoon ground cinnamon

- 1/4 cup water

Instructions:

1. Preheat oven to 350°F (175°C).

2. In a bowl, mix the chopped nuts, raisins, and cinnamon.

3. Stuff the cored apples with the nut mixture.

4. Place the stuffed apples in a baking dish and add water to the bottom of the dish.

5. Bake for 30-35 minutes, or until the apples are tender.

Frozen Banana Pops

Ingredients:

- 4 bananas, peeled and halved

- 8 wooden popsicle sticks

- 1/2 cup dark chocolate, melted

- Toppings: crushed nuts, shredded coconut, or sprinkles

Instructions:

1. Insert a popsicle stick into each banana half.

2. Dip the bananas in melted dark chocolate, then roll in your choice of toppings.

3. Place the banana pops on a parchment-lined tray and freeze for at least 2 hours.

Ingredients:

- 1 large round slice of watermelon, about 1-inch thick

- 1/2 cup Greek yogurt

- Mixed fresh berries (strawberries, blueberries, raspberries)

- A handful of mint leaves

- Honey or balsamic glaze for drizzling (optional)

Instructions:

1. Spread Greek yogurt over the watermelon slice.

2. Arrange the mixed berries on top of the yogurt.

3. Garnish with mint leaves and drizzle with honey or balsamic glaze if desired.

4. Cut into wedges and serve like a pizza.

These fruit-based desserts are not only refreshing and delicious but also offer a guilt-free way to indulge in something sweet while keeping your metabolism in mind.

Healthy Baked Goods Desserts

Healthy Baked Goods Desserts and Treats for Guilt-Free Indulgence

Indulging in healthy baked goods can satisfy your sweet cravings while keeping your metabolism in mind. Some recipes for guilt-free desserts and treats:

Almond Flour Banana Bread

Ingredients:

- 2 ripe bananas, mashed

- 2 cups almond flour

- 3 eggs

- 1/4 cup honey or maple syrup

- 1 teaspoon baking soda

- 1 teaspoon vanilla extract

- 1/2 teaspoon cinnamon

- Pinch of salt

Instructions:

1. Preheat oven to 350°F (175°C).

2. In a bowl, mix mashed bananas, eggs, honey, and vanilla extract.

3. Add almond flour, baking soda, cinnamon, and salt. Mix until well combined.

4. Pour the batter inside a greased loaf pan.

5. Bake for about 45-50 minutes, until a toothpick inserted into the center comes out clean.

Ingredients:

- 1 cup rolled oats

- 3/4 cup whole wheat flour

- 1/2 cup unsweetened applesauce

- 1/4 cup honey or maple syrup

- 1 egg

- 1 teaspoon vanilla extract

- 1/2 teaspoon baking soda

- 1/2 cup dark chocolate chips

- Pinch of salt

Instructions:

1. Preheat oven to 350°F (175°C).

2. In a bowl, mix oats, flour, baking soda, and salt.

3. In another bowl, whisk together applesauce, honey, egg, and vanilla extract.

4. Combine wet and dry ingredients. Fold in chocolate chips.

5. Drop spoonfuls of dough onto a baking sheet.

6. Bake for 10-12 minutes, or until edges are golden brown.

Carrot Cake Muffins

Ingredients:

- 1 1/2 cups whole wheat flour

- 1/2 cup grated carrots

- 1/3 cup unsweetened applesauce

- 1/3 cup honey or maple syrup

- 2 eggs

- 1/4 cup milk (almond, oat, or cow's)

- 1 teaspoon baking powder

- 1/2 teaspoon baking soda

- 1 teaspoon cinnamon

- 1/4 teaspoon nutmeg

- Pinch of salt

Instructions:

1. Preheat oven to 350°F (175°C).

2. In a bowl, mix flour, baking powder, baking soda, cinnamon, nutmeg, and salt.

3. In another bowl, whisk together applesauce, honey, eggs, and milk.

4. Combine wet and dry ingredients. Fold in grated carrots.

5. Fill muffin cups with the batter.

6. Bake for about 20-25 minutes, until a toothpick inserted into the center comes out clean.

Ingredients:

- 2 ripe bananas, mashed

- 1/3 cup melted coconut oil

- 1/2 cup honey or maple syrup

- 2 eggs

- 1/4 cup milk or almond milk

- 1 teaspoon vanilla extract

- 1 teaspoon baking soda

- 1/2 teaspoon salt

- 1/2 teaspoon ground cinnamon

- 1 3/4 cups whole wheat flour

Instructions:

1. Preheat oven to 325°F (165°C). Grease a 9x5 inch loaf pan.

2. In a large bowl, mix mashed bananas, coconut oil or applesauce, honey or maple syrup, eggs, milk, and vanilla extract.

3. Add baking soda, salt, and cinnamon. Stir all whole wheat flour until just combined.

4. Pour batter into the prepared loaf pan.

5. Bake for about 55-60 minutes, until a toothpick inserted into the center comes out clean.

Almond Flour Chocolate Chip Cookies

Ingredients:

- 2 1/2 cups almond flour

- 1/2 teaspoon baking soda

- 1/4 teaspoon salt

- 1/4 cup coconut oil, melted

- 1/4 cup maple syrup or honey

- 1 egg

- 1 teaspoon vanilla extract

- 1/2 cup dark chocolate chips

Instructions:

1. Preheat oven to 350°F (175°C). Line a bake sheet with parchment paper.

2. In a bowl, mix almond flour, baking soda, and salt.

3. Whisk together melted coconut oil, maple syrup or honey, egg, and vanilla extract in another bowl.

4. Combine wet and dry ingredients. Stir in chocolate chips.

5. Drop a tablespoon and size the dough balls onto the prepared baking sheet.

6. Bake for 10-12 minutes, or until edges are golden brown.

DESSERTS AND TREATS FOR GUILT-FREE INDULGENCE

Low-Sugar Sweet Treats

Indulging in low-sugar sweet treats can satisfy your cravings without derailing your metabolic diet. Here are some recipes for desserts and treats that are guilt-free and delicious:

Avocado Chocolate Mousse

Ingredients:

- 2 ripe avocados

- 1/4 cup unsweetened cocoa powder

- 1/4 cup almond milk

- 2-3 tablespoons maple syrup or honey (adjust to taste)

- 1 teaspoon vanilla extract

- Pinch of salt

Instructions:

1. Scoop the avocado flesh into a blender or food processor.

2. Add cocoa powder, almond milk, maple syrup or honey, vanilla extract, and a pinch of salt.

3. Blend until smooth and creamy.

4. leave in the refrigerator to cold for at least 30 minutes before serving.

Almond and Coconut Energy Balls

Ingredients:

- 1 cup almonds

- 1 cup dates, pitted

- 1/2 cup shredded unsweetened coconut

- 1 tablespoon chia seeds

- 1 tablespoon coconut oil

- 1 teaspoon vanilla extract

Instructions:

1. In a food processor, blend almonds until finely ground.

2. Add dates, shredded coconut, chia seeds, coconut oil, and vanilla extract. Blend until the mixture comes together.

3. Roll the mixture into small balls and refrigerate for at least 30 minutes before serving.

Baked Apple Chips

Ingredients:

- 2-3 apples, thinly sliced

- Cinnamon (optional)

1. Instructions:

2. Preheat oven to 200°F (95°C).

3. Arrange apple slices in a single layer on a baking sheet lined with parchment paper.

4. Sprinkle with cinnamon if desired.

5. Bake for 2-3 hours, flipping halfway through, until the apple slices are dried and crispy.

Greek Yogurt and Berry Parfaits

Ingredients:

- 2 cups Greek yogurt

- 1 cup mixed berries (strawberries, blueberries, raspberries)

- 1/4 cup granola (optional)

- Honey or maple syrup (optional)

Instructions:

1. In serving glasses, layer Greek yogurt, berries, and granola.

2. Drizzle with a little honey or maple syrup if desired.

3. Repeat the layers until the glasses are filled.

Peanut Butter and Banana Ice Cream

Ingredients:

- 3 ripe bananas, sliced and frozen

- 2 tablespoons natural peanut butter

- 1 teaspoon vanilla extract

Instructions:

1. Place frozen banana slices in a food processor or high-speed blender.

2. Add peanut butter and vanilla extract.

3. Blend until smooth and creamy, resembling soft-serve ice cream.

4. Serve immediately or freeze for a firmer texture.

These low-sugar sweet treats are perfect for satisfying your sweet tooth while keeping your metabolism in check. Enjoy them as a guilt-free indulgence anytime!

Fruit-Based Desserts

Fruit-based desserts are a wonderful way to satisfy your sweet tooth while keeping things healthy and guilt-free. Here are some delicious recipes that celebrate the natural sweetness of fruits:

Grilled Peaches with Honey and Yogurt

Ingredients:

- 4 ripe peaches, halved and pitted

- 1 tablespoon olive oil

- 1 cup Greek yogurt

- 2 tablespoons honey

- A pinch of cinnamon (optional)

Instructions:

1. Preheat your grill to medium heat.

2. Brush the cut sides of the peaches with olive oil.

3. Place the peaches cut-side down on the grill and cook for 4-5 minutes, or until grill marks appear.

4. Serve the grilled peaches with a dollop of Greek yogurt, a drizzle of honey, and a sprinkle of cinnamon.

Berry and Kiwi Fruit Salad

Ingredients:

- 1 cup strawberries, sliced

- 1 cup blueberries

- 2 kiwis, peeled and sliced

- 1 tablespoon fresh mint, chopped

- 1 tablespoon lime juice

- 1 teaspoon honey (optional)

Instructions:

1. In a large bowl, combine the strawberries, blueberries, and kiwis.

2. In a small bowl, mix lime juice, honey, and chopped mint.

3. Pour the dressing over the fruit salad and gently toss to combine.

Baked Apples with Cinnamon and Nuts

Ingredients:

- 4 apples, cored

- 1/4 cup chopped walnuts or pecans

- 2 tablespoons raisins

- 1 teaspoon ground cinnamon

- 1/4 cup water

Instructions:

1. Preheat oven to 350°F (175°C).

2. In a bowl, mix the chopped nuts, raisins, and cinnamon.

3. Stuff the cored apples with the nut mixture.

4. Place the stuffed apples in a baking dish and add water to the bottom of the dish.

5. Bake for about 30-35 minutes, or until the apples are tender.

Frozen Banana Pops

Ingredients:

- 4 bananas, peeled and halved

- 8 wooden popsicle sticks

- 1/2 cup dark chocolate, melted

- Toppings: crushed nuts, shredded coconut, or sprinkles

Instructions:

1. Insert a popsicle stick into each banana half.

2. Dip the bananas in melted dark chocolate, then roll in your choice of toppings.

3. Place the banana pops on a parchment-lined tray and freeze for at least 2 hours.

Fruit-Based Desserts Healthy Baked Goods

Fruit-based desserts and healthy baked goods offer a delightful way to enjoy guilt-free indulgence. These treats are perfect for satisfying your sweet tooth while adhering to a nutritious dietary plan. Some recipes that

blend the natural sweetness of fruits with wholesome
ingredients:

Blueberry Oatmeal Crumble Bars

Ingredients:

- 2 cups rolled oats

- 1 cup whole wheat flour

- 1/2 cup maple syrup or honey

- 1/2 cup unsweetened applesauce

- 1 teaspoon baking powder

- 1/2 teaspoon cinnamon

- 1/4 teaspoon salt

- 2 cups fresh or frozen blueberries

- 2 tablespoons chia seeds

- 2 tablespoons lemon juice

Instructions:

1. Preheat the oven to 350°F (175°C). Line a 9x9 inch baking pan with parchment paper.

2. In a large bowl, mix oats, flour, half of the maple syrup, applesauce, baking powder, cinnamon, and salt until well combined.

3. Press 2/3 of the oat mixture in the bottom of the prepared pan.

4. In another bowl, toss blueberries with chia seeds, lemon juice, and the remaining maple syrup. Spread the blueberry mixture over the oat layer.

5. Crumble the remaining oat mixture on top of the blueberries.

6. Bake for about 35-40 minutes, or until the top is golden brown. Cool before cutting into bars.

Ingredients:

- 3 cups rolled oats
- 1 teaspoon baking powder
- 2 teaspoons cinnamon
- 1/4 teaspoon salt
- 1 cup unsweetened almond milk
- 2 eggs
- 1/2 cup applesauce
- 1/4 cup maple syrup or honey
- 1 large apple, peeled and diced

Instructions:

1. Preheat the oven to 375°F (190°C). Grease a 12-cup muffin tin.

2. In a large bowl, mix together oats and baking powder, cinnamon, and salt.

3. In another bowl, whisk together almond milk, eggs, applesauce, and maple syrup.

4. Add wet ingredients to the dry ingredients and stir until its mixed. Fold in diced apple.

5. Divide the mixture evenly among the muffin cups.

6. Bake for 25-30 minutes, or until the tops are set and slightly golden. Let cool before serving.

Peach Raspberry Crisp

Ingredients:

- 4 peaches, sliced

- 1 cup raspberries

- 2 tablespoons cornstarch

- 1/3 cup honey or maple syrup

- For the topping:

- 1 cup rolled oats

- 1/2 cup almond flour

- 1/4 cup chopped almonds or walnuts

- 1/4 cup melted coconut oil

- 1/4 cup maple syrup or honey

- 1/2 teaspoon cinnamon

Instructions:

1. Preheat the oven to 350°F (175°C).

2. In a large bowl, toss peaches and raspberries with cornstarch and honey. Transfer to a baking dish.

3. In another bowl, mix oats, almond flour, nuts, coconut oil, maple syrup, and cinnamon until crumbly.

4. Sprinkle the oat mixture over the fruit.

5. Bake for about 30-35 minutes, or until the fruit is bubbly and the topping is golden brown.

These fruit-based desserts and healthy baked goods are not only delicious but also packed with nutrients, making them perfect for a guilt-free indulgence. Enjoy these treats that satisfy your sweet cravings while supporting your overall health.

WEEKLY MEAL PLANS AND SHOPPING LISTS

Sample 7-Day Metabolism Diet Meal Plan

Creating a 7-day metabolism diet meal plan can help you organize your meals and ensure you're getting a balanced intake of nutrients to support your metabolic health. Sample meal plan to get you started:

Day 1:

- **Breakfast**: Green Metabolism Booster Smoothie
- **Lunch**: Grilled Chicken and Veggie Pita
- **Snack**: Carrot and Cucumber Sticks with Hummus
- **Dinner**: Spicy Turkey and Green Bean Skillet

Day 2:

- **Breakfast**: Berry Almond Overnight Oats

- **Lunch**: Turkey Avocado Wrap

- **Snack**: Apple Slices with Almond Butter

- **Dinner**: Baked Salmon with Dill Yogurt Sauce and Quinoa

Day 3:

- **Breakfast**: Banana Nut Porridge

- **Lunch**: Chickpea and Sweet Potato Curry

- **Snack**: Greek Yogurt with Mixed Berries

- **Dinner**: Lemon Garlic Tilapia with Steamed Broccoli

Day 4:

- **Breakfast**: Whole Wheat Banana Muffins

- **Lunch**: Spinach and Feta Stuffed Chicken Breast with a Side Salad

- **Snack**: Baked Apple Chips

- **Dinner**: Beef and Asparagus Skillet

- **Breakfast**: Avocado Toast with Poached Egg on Whole Grain Bread

- **Lunch**: Quinoa Stuffed Bell Peppers

- **Snack**: Cucumber Slices with Guacamole

- **Dinner**: Grilled Shrimp and Vegetable Skewers

Day 6:

- **Breakfast**: Oatmeal with Sliced Almonds and Blueberries

- **Lunch**: Lentil Soup with a Side of Whole Grain Bread

- **Snack**: Almond and Coconut Energy Balls

- **Dinner**: Chicken and Cauliflower Fried "Rice"

Day 7:

- **Breakfast**: Smoothie Bowl with Spinach, Banana, and Chia Seeds

- **Lunch**: Turkey, Apple, and Brie Panini

- **Snack**: Bell Pepper Nachos

- **Dinner**: Zucchini Noodles with Tomato Sauce and Meatballs

Remember to drink plenty of water throughout the day and adjust portion sizes and snack options based on your individual energy needs and dietary preferences. This meal plan is a starting point, and you can modify it to include your favorite metabolic-friendly foods and recipes.

Customizable Meal Plan Templates

Creating customizable meal plan templates can help you stay organized and ensure you're getting a balanced diet that supports your metabolic health. Here's a basic template you can use and modify according to your preferences and nutritional needs:

Daily Meal Plan Template:

- **Breakfast**: [Protein source] + [Whole grain or fruit] + [Healthy fat]

Example: Scrambled eggs + Whole grain toast + Avocado slices

- **Mid-Morning Snack**: [Fruit or vegetable] + [Protein or healthy fat]

Example: Apple slices + Almond butter

- **Lunch**: [Lean protein] + [Whole grain or starchy vegetable] + [non-starchy vegetables] + [Healthy fat]

Example: Grilled chicken breast + Quinoa + Steamed broccoli + Olive oil dressing

- **Afternoon Snack**: [Protein or healthy fat] + [Fruit or vegetable]

Example: Greek yogurt + Mixed berries

- **Dinner**: [Lean protein] + [Whole grain or starchy vegetable] + [non-starchy vegetables] + [Healthy fat]

Example: Baked salmon + Sweet potato + Roasted asparagus + A drizzle of coconut oil

- **Evening Snack** (optional): [Light protein or healthy fat]

Example: Cottage cheese or a handful of nuts

Weekly Meal Plan Template:

Monday:

- Breakfast: [Your choice]

- Mid-Morning Snack: [Your choice]

- Lunch: [Your choice]

- Afternoon Snack: [Your choice]

- Dinner: [Your choice]

Tuesday:

- Breakfast: [Your choice]

- Mid-Morning Snack: [Your choice]

- Lunch: [Your choice]

- Afternoon Snack: [Your choice]

- Dinner: [Your choice]

Wednesday:

- Breakfast: [Your choice]

- Mid-Morning Snack: [Your choice]

- Lunch: [Your choice]

- Afternoon Snack: [Your choice]

- Dinner: [Your choice]

Thursday:

- Breakfast: [Your choice]

- Mid-Morning Snack: [Your choice]

* Lunch: [Your choice]

* Afternoon Snack: [Your choice]

* Dinner: [Your choice]

Friday:

* Breakfast: [Your choice]

* Mid-Morning Snack: [Your choice]

* Lunch: [Your choice]

* Afternoon Snack: [Your choice]

* Dinner: [Your choice]

Saturday:

* Breakfast: [Your choice]

* Mid-Morning Snack: [Your choice]

* Lunch: [Your choice]

* Afternoon Snack: [Your choice]

- Dinner: [Your choice]

Sunday:

- Breakfast: [Your choice]

- Mid-Morning Snack: [Your choice]

- Lunch: [Your choice]

- Afternoon Snack: [Your choice]

- Dinner: [Your choice]

Notes:

- Feel free to swap meals and snacks as needed.

- Adjust portion sizes based on your individual calorie and nutrient requirements.

- Include a variety of foods throughout the week to ensure a balanced intake of nutrients.

- This template is designed to be flexible, allowing you to mix and match meals and snacks to suit your tastes and dietary needs while maintaining a focus on metabolic health.

YOUR OBSERVATION

Your Observation:

Note:

Shopping Lists for Efficient Grocery Shopping

Creating a shopping list is essential for efficient grocery shopping, especially when following a metabolic diet. Here's a sample shopping list that covers various food groups and can be customized based on your meal plan:

Protein Sources:

- Chicken breast

- Turkey breast

- Lean beef (e.g., sirloin)

- Salmon

- Tuna (canned in water)

- Eggs

- Greek yogurt

- Cottage cheese

- Tofu

- Tempeh

Whole Grains and Starchy Vegetables:

- Quinoa

- Brown rice

- Whole wheat pasta

- Oats

- Sweet potatoes

- Butternut squash

Non-Starchy Vegetables:

- Broccoli

- Spinach

- Kale

- Bell peppers

- Asparagus

- Zucchini

- Cucumbers

- Tomatoes

- Cauliflower

- Green beans

Fruits:

- Apples

- Berries (strawberries, blueberries, raspberries)

- Bananas

- Oranges

- Kiwi

- Grapes

- Pineapple

Healthy Fats:

- Avocados

- Olive oil

- Coconut oil

- Nuts (almonds, walnuts, cashews)

- Seeds (chia, flaxseed, pumpkin seeds)

- Nut butters (almond butter, peanut butter)

Dairy or Dairy Alternatives:

- Almond milk

- Oat milk

- Unsweetened yogurt

- Cheese (feta, goat cheese, Parmesan)

Miscellaneous:

- Herbs and spices (basil, oregano, cinnamon, cumin)

- Vinegars (apple cider vinegar, balsamic vinegar)

- Low-sodium soy sauce or tamari

- Honey or maple syrup

- Whole grain bread or wraps

- Hummus

- Canned beans (black beans, chickpeas)

Remember to adjust the quantities based on your meal plan and the number of people you're shopping for. Having a well-organized shopping list can help you save time, reduce food waste, and ensure you have all the ingredients you need for your metabolic diet meals.

Mindful Eating and Portion Control

Mindful eating and portion control are essential components for success in any diet plan, including a metabolic diet. Here are some tips to help you practice mindful eating and manage your portions:

Mindful Eating:

- Pay Attention to Your Body: Pay attention to indicators associated with hunger and fullness. Eat when you're hungry and stop when you're comfortably full.

- Eat Slowly: Take your time to chew your food thoroughly and enjoy each bite. This allows your body to recognize when it's full and can prevent overeating.

- Limit Distractions: Avoid eating in front of the TV, computer, or while on your phone. Focus on your meal and the experience of eating.

- Savor Your Food: Notice the flavors, textures, and aromas of your food. Appreciating your food can enhance satisfaction and help you eat less.

- Practice Gratitude: Before you eat, take a moment to be thankful for your food and the nourishment it provides.

Portion Control:

- Use Smaller Plates: Smaller dishes naturally lead to smaller portions, which can help prevent overeating.

- Measure Your Food: Use measuring cups, spoons, or a food scale to ensure accurate portion sizes, especially for calorie-dense foods like nuts, oils, and cheese.

- Fill Half Your Plate with Vegetables: Non-starchy vegetables are low in calories and high in fiber, helping you feel full with fewer calories.

- Split Meals at Restaurants: Restaurant portions are often larger than necessary. Consider sharing a meal or packing half to take home for later.

- Pre-Portion Snacks: Instead of eating directly from the package, portion out snacks into individual servings to avoid mindless eating.

By incorporating mindful eating and portion control into your daily routine, you can enhance your metabolic health, achieve your weight goals, and develop a healthier relationship with food.

Staying Motivated and Overcoming Challenges

Staying motivated and overcoming challenges are crucial aspects of maintaining a healthy lifestyle and achieving your metabolic health goals. Here are some strategies to help you stay on track:

Set Realistic Goals:

Your long-term objectives should be broken down into more manageable and attainable stages. Celebrating these smaller victories can keep you motivated.

Create a Support System:

Surround yourself with friends, family, or a support group who encourage and support your health journey. Sharing your successes and challenges with others can provide motivation and accountability.

Find Activities You Enjoy:

Find physical activities that you take pleasure in and look forward to participating in. Whether it's walking, dancing, cycling, or yoga, finding joy in exercise can help you stay consistent.

Keep a Food and Exercise Journal:

Tracking your meals and physical activity can help you stay accountable and identify patterns or areas for improvement.

Plan for Setbacks:

Recognize that experiencing failures is a natural and expected part of any endeavor. Instead of getting discouraged, use them as learning opportunities to adjust your plan and keep moving forward.

Reward Yourself:

Celebrate your progress with non-food rewards, such as a new workout outfit, a massage, or a relaxing bath. These rewards can provide extra motivation to reach your goals.

Stay Flexible:

Always open to adjusting your plan as needed. Life can be unpredictable, so being flexible with your routine can help you navigate challenges without derailing your progress.

Practice Self-Compassion:

Kindness and understanding should be shown to oneself at all times, but especially when things are difficult. Remember that progress is not always linear, and it's okay to have ups and downs.

Visualize Success:

Take a few minutes out of each day to see yourself doing the things you have set out to do. This mental visualization has the potential to increase both your motivation and your self-confidence.

Educate Yourself:

Continue learning about metabolic health and wellness. Understanding the benefits of your efforts can reinforce your commitment to a healthy lifestyle.

By implementing these strategies, you can stay motivated, overcome challenges, and make lasting changes that support your metabolic health.

Adjusting the Metabolism Diet for Your Needs

Adjusting the metabolism diet to fit your individual needs is essential for long-term success and overall health. Here are some tips for personalizing your diet:

1. Identify Your Goals

- Determine your specific goals, whether it's weight loss, improved energy levels, better blood sugar control, or overall health. Tailor your diet to support these objectives.

2. Listen to Your Body

- Pay attention to how to make different foods you like. If certain foods cause discomfort or don't seem to support your goals, consider eliminating or reducing them in your diet.

3. Consider Your Activity Level

•   If you're very active, you may need to increase your intake of complex carbohydrates and protein to fuel your workouts and support muscle recovery.

4. Manage Portion Sizes

•   Adjust portion sizes based on your calorie needs, which can vary depending on factors like age, sex, weight, and activity level.

5. Incorporate Variety

•   Ensure a diverse intake of foods to get a wide range of nutrients. Rotate your protein sources, vegetables, fruits, and whole grains to keep your meals interesting and nutritionally balanced.

6. Focus on Nutrient Density

•   Choose foods that are high in nutrients but lower in calories to support your metabolism without excess energy intake.

7. Stay Hydrated

• Proper hydration is crucial for metabolic processes. Adjust your fluid intake based on your activity level, climate, and individual needs.

8. Monitor Your Progress

- Regularly assess your progress toward your goals and make adjustments as needed. This might involve tweaking your macronutrient ratios, changing your meal timing, or modifying your food choices.

9. Seek Professional Guidance

- Consider consulting with a registered dietitian or nutritionist who can provide personalized advice and help you make informed adjustments to your diet.

10. Be Flexible

- Life circumstances and health needs can change over time. Be open to adjusting your diet as needed to continue supporting your metabolic health.

By customizing the metabolism diet to suit your individual needs, you can create a sustainable eating plan that supports your health goals and fits your lifestyle.

CONCLUSION

This book serves as a comprehensive guide to kick-starting and maintaining a healthy metabolism through thoughtful meal preparation and nutrient-rich recipes. By embracing the principles outlined in this book, you can simplify your dietary routine while ensuring that your body receives the fuel it needs to thrive.

The recipes and meal plans provided are designed to cater to a variety of tastes and preferences, making it easier for you to integrate them into your daily life. The emphasis on whole, unprocessed foods, balanced macronutrients, and portion control will not only support your metabolic health but also contribute to your overall well-being.

As you embark on this journey, remember that consistency is key. Meal prepping can streamline your eating habits, reduce decision fatigue, and help you stay on track with your health goals. Embrace the process, and allow yourself to be flexible and adjust as needed based on your body's response and your evolving needs.

"The Complete Easy Metabolism Diet Meal Prep: 2024 Edition" is more than just a cookbook; it's a tool to empower you to take control of your health, one meal at a time. Let this book be your guide to a more energetic, vibrant, and balanced life.

Reflecting on Your Metabolic Diet Journey

Reflecting on your metabolic diet journey is a crucial step in understanding your progress, learning from your experiences, and planning for continued success. Here are some key points to consider during your reflection:

Assess Your Progress:

- **Physical Changes**: Have you noticed improvements in your weight, energy levels, or overall health? Reflect on any positive changes you've experienced since starting the metabolic diet.

- **Emotional Well-being**: Consider how your diet has impacted your mood and mental health. Have you felt more balanced, less stressed, or more confident?

Evaluate Your Eating Habits:

- **Consistency**: How consistent have you been with following the metabolic diet? Identify any patterns or triggers that may have led to deviations from your plan.

- **Challenges**: Reflect on the challenges you've faced, such as cravings, social events, or time constraints. How did you handle these obstacles, and what can you learn from them?

- **Favorites**: Identify your favorite meals and snacks from the diet. Consider how you can incorporate these into your long-term eating plan.

- **Physical Activity**: How has your exercise routine complemented your metabolic diet? Reflect on the types and frequency of physical activities you've engaged in.

- **Mindfulness and Stress Management**: Consider any stress-reduction techniques or mindfulness practices you've adopted and their impact on your overall well-being.

Plan for the Future:

- **Adjustments**: Based on your reflection, identify any adjustments you might need to make to your diet or lifestyle to continue supporting your metabolic health.

- **Goals**: Set new goals or refine existing ones to keep you motivated and focused on your health journey.

- **Support System**: Think about the support you've received and how you can continue to leverage this support or seek additional resources as needed.

Celebrate Your Successes:

- Take a moment to celebrate your achievements, no matter how big or small. Acknowledge the effort you've put into your metabolic diet journey and the positive changes you've made.

Reflecting on your metabolic diet journey allows you to take stock of where you've been, where you are, and where you're headed. Use this reflection as a tool to empower yourself to continue making choices that support your health and well-being.

Continuing Your Path to Metabolic Health

Continuing your path to metabolic health requires a long-term commitment to maintaining a balanced diet, staying active, and making mindful lifestyle choices. Here are some tips to help you stay on track and keep progressing toward your goals:

Stay Informed

Keep learning about metabolic health and nutrition. Staying informed will help you make better choices and adapt your diet as new research emerges.

Set Realistic Goals

Set achievable goals that are specific, measurable, and time-bound. Regularly review and adjust your goals as needed.

Plan Your Meals

Continue meal planning and prepping to ensure you have healthy options readily available. This will help you stay consistent and avoid impulsive, less healthy choices.

Monitor Your Progress

Keep track of your dietary intake, physical activity, and any changes in your health metrics. Regular monitoring can help you identify areas for improvement and celebrate your successes.

Stay Active

Incorporate regular physical activity into your routine. Find activities you enjoy, whether it's walking, cycling, yoga, or strength training.

Listen to Your Body

Pay attention to how different foods and activities make you feel. Adjust your diet and lifestyle based on your body's signals.

Manage Stress

Practice stress-reducing techniques such as mindfulness, meditation, or deep breathing exercises. Managing stress is crucial for maintaining metabolic health.

Stay Hydrated

Drink plenty of water throughout the day to support your body's metabolic processes.

Get Adequate Sleep

Prioritize getting enough quality sleep each night. Sleep is essential for metabolic health and overall well-being.

Seek Support

Surround yourself with supportive friends, family, or a community that shares your health goals. Consider working with a healthcare professional, such as a dietitian or a personal trainer, for personalized guidance.

Be Flexible

Life can be unpredictable, so be prepared to adapt your plans as needed. Flexibility is key to maintaining a healthy lifestyle in the long term.

Celebrate Your Achievements

Acknowledge your hard work and progress, no matter how small. Celebrating your achievements can keep you motivated and focused on your journey.

Continuing your path to metabolic health is a lifelong journey. By staying committed, adaptable, and positive, you can achieve and maintain a healthy metabolism and enjoy a vibrant, fulfilling life.

Substitutions and Swaps for Common Ingredients

Making substitutions and swaps for common ingredients can help you maintain a balanced and varied diet while catering to dietary restrictions, preferences, or health goals. Here are some common ingredient substitutions:

Dairy Substitutes:

Milk: Replace cow's milk with almond, oat, soy, or coconut milk.

Butter: Use coconut oil, olive oil, or avocado as a substitute in baking and cooking.

Cheese: Opt for nutritional yeast, cashew cheese, or vegan cheese alternatives.

Yogurt: Use coconut yogurt, almond milk yogurt, or soy yogurt for a dairy-free option.

Protein Substitutes:

Meat: Replace with beans, lentils, tofu, tempeh, or seitan for plant-based protein sources.

Eggs: Use flaxseed meal or chia seeds mixed with water, applesauce, mashed banana, or commercial egg replacers in baking.

Sweetener Substitutes:

Sugar: Substitute with honey, maple syrup, agave nectar, or stevia for natural sweetness.

Brown Sugar: Use coconut sugar or a mix of white sugar and molasses as alternatives.

Flour Substitutes:

All-Purpose Flour: Replace with whole wheat flour, almond flour, coconut flour, or oat flour for different nutritional profiles and dietary needs.

Breadcrumbs: Use rolled oats, almond meal, or crushed nuts for a gluten-free alternative.

Oil and Fat Substitutes:

Vegetable Oil: Substitute with healthier oils like olive oil, avocado oil, or coconut oil.

Mayonnaise: Use mashed avocado or Greek yogurt as a healthier spread or dressing base.

Other Common Substitutions:

Pasta: Opt for whole-grain pasta, lentil pasta, zucchini noodles, or spaghetti squash for lower-carb alternatives.

Rice: Replace white rice with brown rice, quinoa, cauliflower rice, or farro for added nutrients and fiber.

Soy Sauce: Use tamari or coconut for gluten-free or soy-free alternatives.

Cream: Substitute with coconut milk or cashew cream in soups and sauces.

When making substitutions, it's important to consider how the swap may affect the flavor, texture, and nutritional content of the dish. Experimenting with different alternatives can help you find the best options for your dietary needs and preferences